THROMBOCYTOPENIA

Edited by **Pankaj Abrol**

Thrombocytopenia
http://dx.doi.org/10.5772/intechopen.69080
Edited by Pankaj Abrol

Contributors

Klara Gadó, Luzia De-Oliveira-Pinto, Tamiris Azamor Da Costa Barros, Jen Chin Wang, Thi Huong Nguyen, Gabriela Droc, Pankaj Abrol

Published by InTech
Janeza Trdine 9, 51000 Rijeka, Croatia

Publishing Process Manager Marina Dusevic
Technical Editor SPi Global
Cover InTech Design team

First published March, 2018
Printed in Croatia
Legal deposit, Croatia: National and University Library in Zagreb

Additional hard copies can be obtained from orders@intechopen.com

Thrombocytopenia, Edited by Pankaj Abrol
p. cm.
Print ISBN 978-953-51-3875-4
Online ISBN 978-953-51-3876-1

For EU product safety concerns:
IN TECH d.o.o., Prolaz Marije Krucifikse Kozulić 3, 51000 Rijeka, Croatia,
info@intechopen.com or visit our website at intechopen.com.

Meet the editor

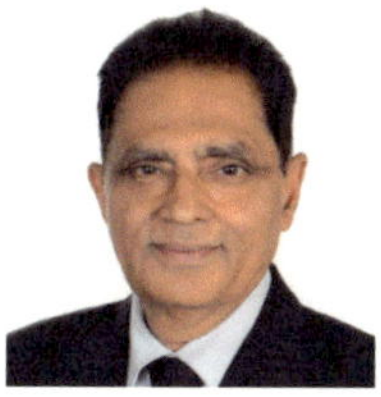

Dr. Pankaj Abrol is presently a Professor and the Head of the Department of Pediatrics, SGT Medical College Hospital & Research Institute, Gurgaon, India. He is a former Senior Professor and the Head of Pediatrics-II in Postgraduate Institute of Medical Sciences, Rohtak, where he was a Chief of Pediatric Hematology and Oncology in charge of Thalassemia and Hemophilia Day Care Centers. He established the Pediatric Cancer Unit after being trained at the Tata Memorial Hospital, Mumbai, India. He received his MBBS and MD degrees in Pediatrics from the Institute of Medical Sciences, Banaras Hindu University, Varanasi. He is a resource person for Pediatric Oncology, Thalassemia and Hemophilia at the state and national levels. He has published many research papers and authored many chapters in textbooks. He is a reviewer for various journals in the field of Pediatrics and Pediatric Hematology and Oncology. His exemplary services in the field of Pediatrics and Pediatric Hematology Oncology won him a fellowship from the Indian Academy of Pediatrics "FIAP." He has more than 34 years of teaching experience producing many graduates and postgraduates.

Contents

Preface

Blood is a vital fluid in the human body. It has important cells and plasma as its constituents. One important type of cell is "platelet" or thrombocyte. Platelet has various functions such as coagulation and immunology. The number and quality of platelet cells should be optimum for normal hemostasis. Low platelet count or "thrombocytopenia" interferes with the normal equilibrium. It gives me immense pleasure to edit a book on this topic. We do not have enough books/publications to do justice to this important topic. Only the optimum management of this condition can affect the clinical outcome of patients with thrombocytopenia.

Science is constantly progressing and it never stops. New concepts are always forthcoming. This book covers the new literature and is quite up to date. State-of-the-art chapters have been written by the experienced authors.

Dengue is a common disease in various parts of the world. Patients can recover without any complication, but some develop severe thrombocytopenia. Immunopathogenesis of thrombocytopenia in patients with dengue must be well understood to provide adequate management. This book provides details about this aspect of thrombocytopenia. It also provides comprehensive studies about thrombocytopenia in antiphospholipid syndrome (APS) and management of thrombocytopenia in APS. The latest literature has been provided by the authors. In these days of organ transplantation, one should know the mechanism of thrombocytopenia in patients with chronic liver diseases and liver transplant, which is discussed in light of the latest references. Interferon had been a primary therapy for diseases such as HCV, CML, multiple sclerosis, etc., for quite a long time. Interferon can induce thrombotic microangiopathy in many such patients. This observation along with later studies has helped us to understand immunobiology and its consequent application in immunomodulating therapeutics. This book "Thrombocytopenia" shall provide the latest literature on the topic. Heparin, an anticoagulant used quite often, is also associated with thrombocytopenia. The mechanism of thrombocytopenia, whether unfractionated or LMWH, has to be used. Such studies with latest observations have been included in a chapter on this topic.

Thus, it can be fairly concluded that the book "Thrombocytopenia" covers important topics and provides a good insight into the latest literature about the topic. I sincerely hope it will serve as a guide to students, scientists and clinicians working in the field.

Dr. Pankaj Abrol
Professor and Head
Department of Pediatrics
SGT Medical College Hospital & Research Institute
Gurgaon (Haryana), India

Chapter 1

Introductory Chapter: Thrombocytopenia

Pankaj Abrol

Additional information is available at the end of the chapter

http://dx.doi.org/10.5772/intechopen.74118

1. Thrombocytopenia

Normal platelet count in blood is 150,000–450,000/μL. Decreased platelet cell count (<150,000/μL) is called "**Thrombocytopenia**." Higher than normal platelet count is called "**Thrombocytosis**." Thrombocytopenia may be an incidental finding or patient can present with fatal hemorrhages. The causes of thrombocytopenia may vary from decreased production to increased destruction.

Platelets or thrombocytes are important blood cells like red and white cells. These are non-nucleated cellular fragments produced by megakaryocytes in bone marrow. On maturity of megakaryocytes, cytoplasm budding occurs releasing large number of platelets. Platelet production is controlled by a growth factor called "**Thrombopoietin (TPO)**." Life span of platelets is 10–14 days. Their count and functional status, both are important to maintain normal hemostasis. Bleeding does not occur usually if platelet count is >100,000/μL. Most of the patients bleed when platelet count falls to <10,000–20,000/μL. They can bleed at higher counts if there is associated functional defect with/without additional coagulation disorder.

Platelet surface has receptors for adhesive proteins like von Willebrand factor (VWF), fibrinogen, thrombin, collagen, and adenosine diphosphate (ADP). After tissue trauma, platelet adhesion occurs, activating platelets and forming platelet plug. This initiates coagulation process followed by clot retraction mediated by platelet contractile proteins and cytoskeleton.

Whenever low platelet count is reported in an asymptomatic patient, one must exclude pseudothrombocytopenia—a condition caused by the aggregation of platelets and resulting in false low count of platelets. Repeating the count along with careful look at peripheral smear can exclude this condition. Another cause of apparent thrombocytopenia is hypothermia. Platelets get transiently sequestrated in spleen, liver, and other organs in hypothermic patients. On rewarming, the platelets return to circulation. This phenomenon is also observed in cardiac patients undergoing surgery with hypothermic perfusion.

All patients having thrombocytopenia do not bleed. Etiology of thrombocytopenia is varied. It can be an incidental finding when patient is being investigated as routine health check-up or for some other disease. The patient with thrombocytopenia can be healthy looking, very sick looking as in sepsis or may be in terminal stages of life as in leukemia.

1.1. Immune thrombocytopenic purpura (ITP)

Major cause of acquired thrombocytopenia in childhood is the increased platelet destruction, which can be due to immune or nonimmune causes. One such important immune cause is immune thrombocytopenia which is also called as **immune thrombocytopenic purpura (ITP)**. It is the most common hematological autoimmune disorder. Antibodies produced target the membranes of platelet for accelerated destruction by phagocytes of reticuloendothelial cells, especially those of spleen. After binding of antibodies to platelet surface, circulating antibody-coated platelets are recognized by the Fc receptor on splenic macrophages, ingested and destroyed. The inhibition of megakaryopoiesis also contributes to thrombocytopenia. Usual clinical presentation of acute ITP is in 1–4 year-old child. There may be a history of preceding viral infection, 1–4 weeks before the onset of symptoms. There is a sudden onset of bleeding as generalized petechiae and purpura in otherwise healthy looking child. Gums and mucus membrane may be involved if associated with profound thrombocytopenia (platelet count <10,000/μL). About 80% of children with ITP have platelet count <20,000/μL. Severe bleeding is still rare. Some patients have still lower count <10,000/μL. Peripheral smear may show large platelets reflecting increased platelet turn over. Bone marrow examination is indicated in the presence of abnormal WBC count and unexplained anemia. Many patients with acute ITP have mild symptoms—petechiae and purpura. Treatment causes early rise of platelet count to safe level of >20,000/μL. Treatment options are: (1) No therapy in mild symptoms. (2) intravenous immunoglobulin (IVIG) 0.8–1.0 g/kg for 1–2 days. Response occurs in 95% patients in 48 hours. It is expensive and time consuming therapy. Patient may have headache and vomiting, indicating IVIG-induced aseptic meningitis. (3) Prednisolone therapy (1–4 mg/kg) usually for short periods until platelet count rises to >20,000/μL. This avoids the long-term side effects of corticosteroids use, like growth failure, osteoporosis, and hypertension. (4) Intravenous anti-D therapy in Rh positive patients. Intravenous anti-D therapy, at the dose of 50–75 μg/kg increases platelet count to >20,000/μL in 80–90% of patients in 48–72 hours. It induces mild hemolytic anemia. It gets bound to Rh positive RBC's, the complex binds to macrophage Fc receptors and interferes with platelet destruction thus raising platelet count [1]. Anti-D is not effective in Rh negative patients. Rarely, it may cause life-threatening intravascular hemolysis. It costs less and also has lesser side effects compared to IVIG. In 20% of patients of ITP, thrombocytopenia is persistent for more than 12 months. These patients are diagnosed as chronic ITP. In such patients, evaluation should be done for diseases like SLE, HIV, von Willebrand disease etc. Splenectomy is the best intervention for long-term results in chronic ITP [2] of such children. Medical therapy with the drugs such as IVIG, steroids, and anti-D used in acute ITP are also useful. Rituximab [3] monoclonal antibody directed against CD 20, has also shown good results. Four weekly doses of 375 mg/m^2 are given. Up to 60% of cases may respond. Thrombopoietic agents such as romiplostim [4, 5] and eltrombopag [6, 7] are also now approved by FDA to treat chronic ITP in adults.

1.2. Neonatal alloimmune thrombocytopenia (NAIT)

It is characterized by transient severe thrombocytopenia. Maternal antibodies are transferred from placenta and are directed against paternally inherited fetal antigens present on fetal/neonatal platelets. Newborn can have severe thrombocytopenia, with platelets as low as 10,000/μL on first day of life. There can be bleeding in the form of petechiae, hematoma, GIT bleed, and ICH. Utero bleeding can result in hydrocephalus, seizures or UID [2]. Immunophenotyping of maternal, paternal, and neonatal platelets along with tests for antiplatelet antibodies in maternal and/or or fetal serum can confirm the diagnosis. Severe NAIT (platelet count <30,000/μL) or severe bleeding can be transfused washed and/or irradiated maternal platelets. IVIG (1 g/kg × 2 days) or methyl prednisolone 2 mg/kg/day can also be used for transient relief [2].

1.3. Drug-induced immune thrombocytopenia

Some drugs cause immune thrombocytopenia more often. Two types of antibodies can be formed: drug dependent and drug independent. With former, thrombocytopenia subsides when drug is stopped. In case of drug independent antibodies, drug-induced antibodies and low platelet count may persist for longer making it difficult to exclude ITP. Treatment starts with stoppage of culprit drug. If drug-induced thrombocytopenia is severe, IVIG or corticosteroids may be used. Platelets may be transfused if life-threatening hemorrhage is anticipated.

1.4. Heparin-induced thrombocytopenia and thrombosis

This syndrome occurs in 1–5% of adults and is less common in children. Usually occurs 5–10 days after administration of heparin but can occur within hours if patient is already sensitized to heparin. Incidence is higher with higher dose of heparin, bovine heparin (compared to porcine heparin), and unfractionated heparin (compared to low molecular weight heparin (LMWH)) [8].

1.5. Thrombotic microangiopathic disorders

It is characterized by thrombocytopenia, capillary thrombosis, and microangiopathic hemolytic anemia. Thrombosis and ischemic necrosis may lead to multiple organ dysfunction and failure. Two important disorders are: thrombotic thrombocytopenic purpura (TTP) and hemolytic uremic syndrome (HUS).

1.6. Thrombotic thrombocytopenic purpura (TTP)

In addition to the above-mentioned triad, TTP patient, usually an adult has fever, renal malfunction, and central nervous changes. Subtle shifting neurological signs such as aphasia, blindness and seizures may be there. Coagulation studies are usually nonconclusive. Blood urea nitrogen and creatinine are at times elevated. Treatment is plasmapheresis. Rituximab, steroids or splenectomy may be indicated in refractory cases.

1.7. Hemolytic uremic syndrome

It is a classical example of community-acquired acute kidney injury in children. Clinical features are common to TTP but are seen usually in young children, whereas TTP is disease of adults (rarely in adolescents). History of enteritis due to toxin producing *Escherichia coli* and *Shigella dysenteriae* precedes renal involvement. Pneumonia causing Pneumococci can also cause HUS. As diagnosis is usually clinical, renal biopsy is rarely needed. Anemia is initially mild but progresses. Platelet count is in the range of 20,000–100,000/μL. Coombs test is usually positive. Renal insufficiency is variable. It can progress to renal failure. With early diagnosis and prompt care, mortality is <5%, another 5% become dialysis dependent, and 30% may have persistent renal insufficiency in diarrhea-associated HUS. Mortality can be >20% in Pneumococci-associated HUS.

1.8. Kasabach-Merritt syndrome

Thrombocytopenia is associated with giant hemangioma of infancy. Hemangioma usually solitary may be present over extremities, neck or trunk. Sometimes hemangioma is retroperitoneal. It usually presents in the initial weeks of life, increases in size, and then regresses. Platelet count may be very low with the evidence of DIC. Mortality is 40%. Surgical removal is effective but sometimes not possible. Radiation therapy, vascular ligation/embolization, glucocorticoid therapy, interferon α, vincristine and propranolol are other alternatives.

1.9. Other causes

Infections like systemic bacterial and fungal infections, acute viral infections (e.g., infectious mononucleosis, dengue, and HIV), immunization with live virus vaccines like MMR, hemophagocytic lymphohistiocytosis, malaria, etc., and procedures such as ECMO, hemodialysis, apheresis, liver transplant, etc., can also be associated with thrombocytopenia by increasing their destruction. Dengue is frequently associated with thrombocytopenia. It occurs because of decreased production as well as increased peripheral destruction. Platelet dysfunction is also associated. Drugs like heparin, quinidine, antibiotics like rifampicin and vancomycin also cause thrombocytopenia. Platelets get trapped in enlarged spleen in splenomegaly, portal hypertension, Gaucher disease, etc., and cause low platelet count.

1.10. Thrombocytopenia caused by impaired platelet production

Patients having thrombocytopenia due to the decreased platelet production are more likely to have severe bleeding than those having low platelet count due to the increased platelet destruction. Common causes of decreased production are:

A. **Hereditary disorders:** Examples are congenital amegakaryocytic thrombocytopenia, thrombocytopenia absent radius (TAR) syndrome, Fanconi anemia, Bernard-Soulier syndrome, May-Hegglin anomaly, Gray platelet syndrome, and Wiskott-Aldrich syndrome etc.

B. **Acquired disorders:** This includes megaloblastic anemia (folic acid and vitamin B12 deficiency), aplastic anemia, myelodysplastic syndrome, sepsis, cytotoxic chemotherapy for malignancy, replacement of platelet precursors in bone marrow by malignant cells—leukemia, neuroblastoma, rhabdomyosarcoma, etc.

Thrombocytopenia is quiet common finding in medical practice and is associated with variety of diseases. It can be a benign disorder as ITP in otherwise healthy child. Same patient can die if his intracranial hemorrhage is not managed properly. Thrombocytopenia can be associated with malignant diseases like leukemia, when daily monitoring of platelet count and proper management becomes essential. A patient of dengue can die of dengue hemorrhagic fever and can also recover completely if thrombocytopenia is managed properly. Thus, it is very important to be aware of thrombocytopenia, so that the affected patients can be adequately managed.

Author details

Pankaj Abrol

Address all correspondence to: abrolpankaj1@gmail.com

Department of Pediatrics, Pediatric Hematologist Oncologist, SGT Medical College Hospital and Research Institute, Gurgaon, Haryana, India

References

[1] Scott JP. Idiopathic Thrombocytopenic purpura. In: Nelson Textbook of Pediatrics. 20th ed. Philadelphia: Elsevier; 2015. pp. 2402-2404

[2] Wilson DB. Acquired platelet defects. In: Nathan and Oski's Hematology and Oncology of Infancy and Childhood. 8th ed. Philadelphia: Elsevier Saunders; 2015. pp. 1076-1102

[3] Hasan A, Michel M, Bussel J. Repeated courses of rituximab in chronic ITP: Three different regimens. American Journal of Hematology. 2009;**84**:661-665

[4] Cersosimo RJ. Romiplastin in chronic immune thrombocytopenic purpura. Clinical Therapeutics. 2009;**9**:1887-1907

[5] Kuter DJ, Rummel M, Boccia R, et al. Romiplostim or standard of care in patients with immune thrombocytopenia. The New England Journal of Medicine. 2010;**363**:1889-1899

[6] Bussel JB, Cheng G, Saleh MN, et al. Eltrombopag for treatment of chronic immune thrombocytopenic purpura. The New England Journal of Medicine. 2007;**357**:2237-2247

[7] McMillan R. The pathogenesis of chronic immune thrombocytopenic purpura. Seminars in Hematology. 2007;**44**:S3-S11

[8] Warkentin TE, Levine MN, Hirsh J, et al. Heparin-induced thrombocytopenia in patients treated with low-molecular-weight heparin or unfractionated heparin. The New England Journal of Medicine. 1995;**18**:1330-1335

Chapter 2

A View of Platelets in Dengue

Tamiris Azamor da Costa Barros and
Luzia Maria de-Oliveira-Pinto

Additional information is available at the end of the chapter

http://dx.doi.org/10.5772/intechopen.73084

Abstract

Platelets were mainly associated with coagulation and hemostasis; however, other biological effects have been attributed to platelets, including angiogenesis, extracellular matrix synthesis, inflammation, and immune response. Dengue virus infection causes 200 million cases of severe flu-like illness annually, escalating to life-threatening hemorrhagic fever or shock syndrome. Some hypotheses are postulated for immunopathogenesis of dengue, including antibody enhancement theory, T-cell activation of cross-reactive memory, and original antigenic sin. All hypotheses, to some extent, induce an overproduction or a skewed profile of cytokine release, giving rise to the term cytokine storm/cytokine tsunami. Although thrombocytopenia is typical of both mild and severe diseases, the mechanism triggering platelet reduction is incompletely understood. In dengue, platelets are one of the major cell populations affected by direct and/or indirect mechanisms of infection. It is common to observe both thrombocytopenia and platelet dysfunction in dengue, both strongly related to the clinical outcome. Thus, platelets are frequently affected in dengue, either for alteration of their own functionality, for "silent transport" of virus, or as an anti-viral immune cell. In this way, we describe some of functional aspects of platelets on dengue, observing circulating mediators, intraplatelet proteins contents, morphology, activation markers, and ability to interact with dengue virus.

Keywords: dengue, platelets, thrombocytopenia, dysfunction of platelets, immunopathogenesis

1. Introduction

As the first cellular components accumulate at sites where there is vascular wall damage, platelets rapidly initiate events such as aggregation, exocytosis of granule constituents, adhesion protein expression, cytokine, and others inflammatory mediator's secretion and directly interact with endothelial cells and immune cells. In addition, they can perform the synthesis of new proteins through their complex post-transcription repertoire for post-activation translation, corroborating the existence of potential biological functions of platelets. In dengue, platelets are one of the major cell populations affected by direct and/or indirect mechanisms of infection.

1.1. An overview of immunopathogenesis of dengue

Dengue is one of the arboviruses transmitted by mosquitoes of the genus *Aedes* in a human-mosquito-human cycle. It is endemic in more than 120 countries, where 50 to 100 million infections occur each year, which correspond to 55% of the world population live at risk of infection. Therefore, dengue has the greatest impact on public health worldwide with higher morbidity, albeit fortunately with low mortality rate [1]. The etiologic agent is the dengue virus (DENV), which has four antigenically distinct viral serotypes, the DENV 1 to 4. DENVs share between 65 and 75% homology in their RNA sequences. As a member of the *Flaviviridae* family, the DENV consists of an envelope formed by a lipid bilayer derived from the endoplasmic reticulum of the host cell into which the envelope (E) and membrane (M) proteins are inserted. The viral particle is spherical in shape and approximately 50 nm in diameter. Below the viral envelope is a nucleocapsid composed of an icosahedral viral capsid formed by the capsid protein (C) and complexed to a single-stranded RNA molecule with positive polarity [2, 3]. Viral RNA DENV is approximately 10.7 Kb and is modified at its 5′ end by the addition of the cap structure but is devoid of the poly-A tail at the 3′ end and has a single open reading frame encoding a protein precursor polyprotein viral infection. This precursor protein is cleaved by both host cell proteases and viral protease, yielding 10 proteins: structural C, pre-Membrane (prM)/ M, E, and nonstructural proteins (NS1, NS2A, NS2B, NS3, NS4A, NS4B, and NS5). The translated structural proteins are incorporated into the viral particles during their maturation, while the nonstructural proteins are involved in the replication and/ or assembly of the virions. The 3′and 5′ noncoding regions are also important for viral replication [4–6].

Dengue fever is generally an acute disease, with a broad spectrum of clinical manifestations ranging from a clinically inapparent infection, an undifferentiated acute febrile illness, dengue fever (DF), to more severe forms, dengue hemorrhagic fever (DHF) and dengue shock syndrome (DSS). The first symptoms of DF and DHF are indistinguishable, but DHF is associated with hemorrhagic manifestations, plasma extravasation, and thrombocytopenia (counts below 150,000 platelets/mm^3). Thrombocytopenia is not necessarily restricted to severe forms of dengue, since it is possible to see small bleeding in mild infections. DSS is distinguished from DHF by the presence of cardiovascular or other organs impairment, which occurs when loss of plasma to interstitial spaces results in shock. In general, DSS is a serious disease, with mortality rates of up to 20%, but may also be less than 1% in places with sufficient resources and with clinical experience [7, 8]. Symptomatic disease typically follows three phases: an initial febrile phase lasting 3 to 7 days; a critical phase around the defervescence during which complications may appear in some patients; and a spontaneous recovery phase [9].

A simplified categorization for the classification of dengue severity was proposed by the World Health Organization (WHO) in 2009 in which DHF and DSS were grouped as severe dengue [1]. This classification was based on a multicenter study that treats the illness as a dynamic and systemic event. The new classification describes three sets of clinical signs and symptoms: (1) Dengue fever without signs of alarm (DF) characterized by nausea, vomiting, rash, myalgia, headache, arthralgia, and positive tourniquet test with no signs bleeding and leukopenia; (2) Dengue fever with warning signals (DFwWS) includes abdominal pain or tenderness, persistent vomiting, fluid accumulation, lethargy, agitation, hepatomegaly (increase > 2 cm), elevated serum transaminases, and decreased platelet count; and (3) Severe Dengue Fever characterized by severe plasma extravasation, leading to shock and fluid accumulation, accompanied by respiratory discomfort, severe bleeding, and involvement of organs such as the liver, central nervous system (with altered consciousness), heart, and other organs. This new classification proved to be more sensitive to the identification of severe forms, reducing the proportion of patients previously unclassifiable, which facilitated the clinical management of patients [10].

Briefly, immunopathogenesis of dengue is postulated by some hypotheses, including antibody enhancement theory [11, 12], T-cell activation of cross-reactive memory, and original antigenic sin [13]. All hypotheses, to some extent, induce an overproduction or a skewed profile of cytokine release, giving rise to the term cytokine storm/cytokine tsunami [14].

The humoral response is mainly directed to the prM, E, and NS1 proteins, whereas in the cases of secondary infection, the response against NS3 and NS5 is observed [15, 16]. It is believed that a primary infection can create effective, lasting protection against reinfection by the same serotype, but triggers short-term cross-protection against the other serotypes [17]. Neutralization of infection by specific antibodies may occur by inhibiting the entry of the virus through its specific receptors into the target cell [18] or by inhibiting viral fusion into the target cell cytoplasm [19]. On the other hand, epidemiological studies suggest that homologous immunity may increase the severity of the disease during a subsequent infection by a heterologous serotype [11]. It is believed that low neutralizing antibodies, those that induce cross-reaction, produced in response to a previous serotype, contribute to the pathogenesis of dengue by promoting the entry of the virus through Fcγ receptors into myeloid cells, a phenomenon known as antibody-dependent infection (ADE) [20].

The role of T cells during dengue infection is still controversial, with studies supporting either an immunoprotective or immunopathological role [21]. Pioneer studies proposed that T cells have a detrimental role during secondary dengue infections in a process termed "original antigenic sin." Based on this theory, cross-reactive T cells generated during primary infection, which recognize secondary-infected DENV serotype with low affinity, are poorly functional but prone to inducing immunopathology [13]. Thus, as cross-reactive memory, T cells are present in increased numbers and have a low activation threshold. They may outcompete their naïve subsets that have high affinity for secondary-infected serotype with an overall detrimental outcome for protective immunity [22]. Collectively, studies showed that dengue infection elicits a broad-specific T cell response that peaks around day 8–10 from fever onset [23, 24]. Dengue-specific CD8+ T cells are present at higher frequencies compared to their CD4+ counterparts and preferentially target nonstructural proteins NS3, NS4b, and NS5, while CD4+ T cells are mainly directed toward the capsid envelope and the secreted protein NS1 [23].

Moreover, studies have demonstrated that high concentrations of circulating cytokines, mainly released by T cells, monocytes, macrophages, and endothelial cells from patients, would be involved in the pathogenesis of dengue [24]. Initially, antiviral mechanisms of innate immune response mediated by interferons (IFNs), mainly produced by dendritic cells (DCs), monocytes, macrophages, and natural killer (NKs) cells, are involved in initial infection control. The antiviral activity of type I IFNs (IFN-α/β) is initiated hours after infection and promotes inhibition of viral replication of infected cells, activation of the antiviral state by uninfected cells, and stimulation of the antiviral activity of the cells NK and CD8+ T lymphocytes [25, 26]. DENV proteins such as NS4B and NS5 have been shown to inhibit IFN-α/-β signaling [27–29]. However, *in vitro* and *in vivo* studies have demonstrated that DENV is capable of activating the production of IFN-α by human plasmacytoid dendritic cells (pDC) [30]. The IFN-γ (or IFN-type II), a cytokine involved with Th1 profile, is produced primarily by T lymphocytes, NK cells, and to a lesser extent by macrophages. The IFN-γ, like other IFNs, has an antiviral effect and promotes increased expression of human leukocyte antigen (HLA) class I and II molecules and stimulates antigen presenting and cytokine production by antigen-presenting cells (APCs) [31]. Kurane et al. reported higher levels of IFN-γ in the serum of patients with DHF and DF compared to healthy subjects, but IFN-γ levels were still higher after defervescence in patients with DHF. According to the authors, these results suggest that IFN-γ would play an important role in infection control; however, high levels of this cytokine after defervescence, together with increased T cell activation, would contribute to the pathogenesis of DHF [32]. TNF-α is another cytokine that appears to play an important role in dengue. TNF-α is produced by mononuclear phagocytes, neutrophils, lymphocytes, and NK cells. The interaction of TNF-α and endothelial cells promotes induction of adhesion molecules, such as intracellular adhesion molecule-1 (ICAM-1), vascular cell adhesion molecule-1 (VCAM-1), and E-selectin (E-CD62), being strongly involved in vascular damage, septic shock, and anti-tumor immunity [31]. In dengue, TNF-α appears to be involved in vascular damage, and authors observed an increased permeability and morphological changes in endothelial cells treated in vitro with TNF-α [33]. Studies have shown elevated plasmatic cytokines in dengue, such as IL-1β, IL-2, IL-4, IL-6, IL-7, IL-8, IL-10, IL-13, and IL-18, transforming growth factor-beta-receptor (TGF-β) [34–40]. Chaturvedi et al. reported that DF patients had higher levels of IFN-γ and IL-2, whereas the majority of DHF patients had IL-4, IL-6, and IL-10 elevation, on the 4th and 8th days of the disease, coinciding with the defervescence phase [41]. Pretreatment of monocytes/macrophages with Th2 profile cytokines (IL-4 or IL-13) increased the susceptibility of these cells to DENV infection [42]. Plasma levels of IL-10 were correlated with thrombocytopenia in dengue patients [34, 43]. High production of TNF-α, IL-1β, IL-12, IL-17, soluble IL-1 receptor type 1 protein (sST2), and tumor necrosis factor-related apoptosis-inducing ligand (sTRAIL), as well as apoptosis in DENV-infected monocyte/macrophages cultures, was also observed. It has been shown, therefore, that beneficial or deleterious biomarkers may be present in dengue, regardless of the severity of the disease [44].

2. Thrombocytopenia and dysfunction of platelets in dengue

Reduced proliferative capacity of hematopoietic cells in bone marrow and/or increased destruction of platelets from peripheral blood are two main events associated with thrombocytopenia

[45–47]. Thrombocytopenia occurs when platelet formation (thrombopoiesis) is insufficient to balance physiological or pathological platelet consumption. Thrombocytopenia may occur in patients with either mild or severe cases of dengue infection and are associated in the early days of dengue infection [1]. The WHO guidelines for 2009 reaffirmed that a rapid decline or platelet count below 150,000/mm^3 of blood are one of the indicators of clinical dengue worsening. Together, the functional disturbance associated with deregulation of the plasma quinine system is related with the immunopathogenesis of dengue [1, 48, 49].

2.1. Thrombocytopenia induced by bone marrow suppression, lysis of megakaryocytes and/or peripheral destruction of platelets

The kinetic observation of platelet counts in dengue patients showed a mild to moderate decrease in the 3rd to the 7th day, a significant decrease on day 4, reaching normal levels in the 8th or 9th day of the disease [50, 51]. Profound thrombocytopenia (nadir platelet count ≤20,000/mm^3) was significantly more likely to detect early warning signs and longer hospital stays, but profound thrombocytopenia was not affected by DENV serotypes, coinfections, and secondary DENV infections [52]. However, a study involving 245 dengue patients showed no relationship between bleeding and platelet count, while 81 nonbleeding patients had a score below 20,000/mm^3 [53]. In contrast, another study involving 225 dengue patients suggested that bleeding occurred more frequently in patients with PT [54]. Most clinical guidelines recommend platelet transfusion in patients with dengue who develop severe bleeding or platelet counts below 10–20,000/mm^3. However, another study confirms that platelet transfusion does not prevent the development of severe bleeding or shorten coagulation time [55], and in severe dengue disease with hemorrhagic manifestations, the need for intensive care was not significantly associated with PT [52].

Previous published data indicated that DENV can induce thrombocytopenia through bone marrow suppression, lysis of megakaryocytes, and/or peripheral destruction of platelets [56]. Three main mechanisms seem to be involved, although partially explained, such as a direct lesion of progenitor cells by DENV, infected stromal cells, and modification of bone marrow regulation [51]. In fact, studies have shown a hypocellularity in bone marrow and inhibition of megakaryocyte maturation [51, 57]. *In vitro* studies using an adventitious reticular cell line, which are bone marrow stromal cells, incubated with DENV found DENV antigens in the perinuclear region of these cells [58]. These interactions lead to a modification in the cytokine profile produced in the bone marrow, as in the case of TGF-β capable of inhibiting the differentiation of multipotent stem cells into megakaryocyte precursor cells, leading to inhibition of the cell differentiation process [59, 60]. Another cytokine, the thrombopoietin (TPO), regulates megakaryocytopoiesis and platelet production specifically through the activation of myeloproliferative leukemia virus oncogene (c-MPL), the TPO receptor [61, 62]. When platelet counts fall, circulating levels of TPO increase and may function as a useful indicator of megakaryocytopoiesis in dengue [63, 64]. Recently, authors showed that mice inoculated with recombinant DENV-envelope protein domain III (DENV-EIII)-suppressed megakaryopoiesis of progenitor cells from murine bone marrow and human cord blood in vitro, similarly to those observed with DENV infection. Additional analyses suggested that autophagy impairment and apoptosis are involved in DENV-EIII-mediated suppression of megakaryopoiesis. Thus, these data suggest that, even without viral replication, the binding of DENV-EIII to the cell surface is sufficient to suppress megakaryopoiesis [65].

Although several aspects of the pathogenesis of thrombocytopenia are still not clearly understood, La Russa and Innis in 1995 demonstrated that DENV-induced bone marrow suppression depressed platelet synthesis [58]. In the same year, Wang et al. found that DENV-2 can bind to human platelets in the presence of virus-specific antibody, proposing an immune-mediated clearance of platelets [66]. No infectious model that mimics DHF/DSS has yet been reported until Huang et al. described that the immunocompetent mice intravenous inoculated with DENV-2 developed transient thrombocytopenia and generate IgG class anti-platelet antibody. This was the first evidence of an association between anti-DENV immune response with cross-reactivity to platelets [67]. Falconar gave a strong contribution when identified a highly avid subclone monoclonal antibody MAb 1G5.4-A1-C3 from DENV-2 NS1 and others anti-NS1 MAbs, which in addition of producing hemorrhage in mice, cross-reacted with human fibrinogen, thrombocytes, and endothelial cells, with known epitopes or active sites on human clotting factors and integrin/adhesin proteins present on these cells [68].

Previous study described a strong association between activation status of platelets and their destruction/depletion from circulation in febrile dengue patients [69]. Peripheral destruction of platelets can occur through the direct interaction of the virus in the platelet, as well as indirectly, since the infection leads to the formation of aggregates platelet-endothelial cells and platelets leukocytes or still to the secretion of anti-platelet antibodies and production of factors detrimental to platelets [56]. During dengue infection, cross-reactivity autoantibodies, including antiplatelet antibodies, are generated. In addition, anti-NS1 antibodies belong to the IgM class cross-react with platelets. This last one has the potential for activation of the cascade complement system, leading to the induction of cell lysis and inhibition of platelet aggregation [70, 71]. Notably, high anti-platelet IgM titers were detected in patients with DHF/DSS compared to DF. In accordance with high titers of IgM, serum from DHF/DSS patients causes more platelet lysis than the DF patient serum [71]. Autoantibodies against endothelial cells and blood coagulation molecules have also been described [72]. In fact, molecular mimicry between platelets, endothelial cells, or blood clotting molecules and NS1, prM, and E may explain the cross-reactivity of anti-NS1, anti-prM, or anti-E antibodies between host proteins and proteins. Cross-reactivity antibodies can cause platelet dysfunction, endothelial cell damage, coagulation deficiencies, and activation of macrophages [73]. In addition, it has been recognized that platelet surface P-Selectin (P-CD62) activates integrins and mediates adhesion, aggregation, and secretion of mediators [74].

Among the soluble factors that play a role in the peripheral destruction of platelets, they include platelet-activating factor (PAF) [75], von Willebrand factor (vWF) [76], TNF-α, IL-1β [35], and IL-10 [34].

Platelet apoptosis and phagocytosis associated with high-serum TPO levels were significantly increased in dengue patients during the early stages of convalescence when compared to the late convalescence phase and in healthy volunteers. These results suggest that the abrupt drop in the number of platelets at the beginning of infection is outweighed by TPO-mediated thrombopoiesis [77]. Another study confirmed that platelets from patients exhibited classic signs of the apoptosis intrinsic pathway that include increased phosphatidylserine exposure, mitochondrial depolarization, and activation of caspase-9 and -3 [78].

2.2. Dysfunction of platelets in dengue

Platelet activation is a phenomenon common during physiological dysbalance, such as damage to blood vessels when in contact with components of the subendothelial matrix (collagen and vWF) [79], virus infections such as DENV and human immunodeficiency virus [80], hypothermia [81], diabetes mellitus [82], and arterial thrombosis [83]. Moreover, some agonists involved in platelet activation include adenosine diphosphate (ADP), thromboxane A_2 (TXA_2), collagen, serotonin, epinephrine, and thrombin [84], in addition to pathogens and toxins [85].

During its activation, the platelets undergo a structural change process, in which the discoid cells undergo modifications in the cytoskeleton, disassembly of a ring of microtubules, resulting in an intermediate spherical shape. Next, actin polymerization and filopodia extension occur, causing the cell to acquire lamellar or dendritic morphology [86]. The major activated platelet receptors on interactions with other cells are glycoprotein GP IIb/IIIa (CD41/CD61) and P-CD62. The CD41/CD61 binds to adhesion proteins that contain the Arginine-Glycine-Asparagine peptide sequence (RGD sequence), thus allowing the pooling and binding of activated platelets to leukocytes and endothelial cells via "bridge molecules," such as fibrinogen [87]. P-selectin is a glycoprotein stored in platelet α-granules that is translocated to the surface and released in suspension during platelet activation [85]. It is the main adhesion molecule responsible for platelet interaction with monocytes [85, 88–90], and circulating platelet-monocyte aggregates have been detected in dengue patients [89, 91]. As for the morphological and physiological profile of the platelets exposed to DENV-2, it was observed that there is platelet activation with increased expression of P-CD62 and fibrinogen binding. For morphological changes related to activation, the authors cited membrane architecture alterations, degranulation, the presence of filopodia, and dilation of the open canalicular system in platelets exposed to DENV-2 [92].

The events related to activation are not restricted to changes in morphology, having consequences in several biological functions developed by the platelets. It is also observed exocytosis of constituents of platelet granules, expression of adhesion proteins, and secretion of cytokines and other immunological mediators [93]. Activated platelets secrete mediators stored or synthesized in their granules, which act on several functions. In addition, during plaquetogenesis, megakaryocytes transfer platelet pre-mRNAs, such as tissue factor (TF, inflammatory mediator, and coagulation regulator) pre-mRNA to platelet, are processed to mature mRNA and translated into biologically active TF [94]. In this way, platelets have a complex post-transcriptional repertoire able to translate new proteins, a phenomenon evidenced in response to activation [95, 96]. Multiple pathways lead to platelet activation, including agonists such as collagen, ADP, TXA_2, epinephrine, serotonin, and thrombin, through interaction with receptors on platelet surface, leading to release of its granular content, increase of intracellular Ca^{2+} levels, and activation of the fibrinogen receptor, αIIbβ3 integrin [97–100]. Studies have been reporting platelet dysfunction in dengue infections. In this context, suppression of platelet aggregation has been shown to occur along with an increased release of beta thromboglobulin (βTG) and Platelet Factor 4 (PF4/CXCL4) during the acute phase of DHF [101]. Assays using mononuclear leukocytes (MNLs) from healthy donors exposed to DENV-1 and 2 release significantly greater amounts of PAF, TXB_2, and Prostaglandin D2 (PGD2) than the donor not exposed to any DENV serotypes [102]. Previous data showed that TXB_2 plasma levels of DHF patients with shock decreased significantly than those of normal controls and DHF patients without shock patients, supposing that failure or inadequate TXB_2 production may eventually lead to shock [103].

In addition to exerting an effector role, platelets influence the production of cytokines by peripheral mononuclear cells. Activated platelets exhibit anti-inflammatory properties related to the CD40 and CD40L interaction, leading to increased IL-10 production and inhibition of TNF-α by monocytes [104]. The authors also verified that the interaction of apoptotic monocytes and platelets regulates the secretion of IL-10 through the recognition of platelet phosphatidylserine. It appears that IL-10 secretion requires only monocyte-platelet contact, but not phagocytosis, indicating that activated and apoptotic platelets aggregate to monocytes during infection [86]. Azeredo et al. found that IL-10 levels were correlated with low platelet counts [34]. Platelets are the major source of TGF-β1 in the human body [105]. One study has shown that circulating levels of TGF-β1 are significantly lower in patients with DHF than in controls [106]. Patients with immune thrombocytopenia have low levels of TGF-β1 in the circulation. However, after therapy to restore normal platelet count, their TGF-β1 levels return to levels found in healthy controls [107].

The innate immune system recognizes infection and changes in cellular homeostasis to initiate responses to clear pathogens and repair tissue damage. Toll-like receptors (TLRs) are part of the innate immune system, key players that modulate the inflammatory response and tumor dynamics. Many investigators have confirmed the expression of TLR1-9 both human and murine platelets [108]. Other major complex involved in these processes is the inflammasome, a multimeric protein complex that activates pro-caspase-1, which then proceeds to cleave multiple substrates including the pro-inflammatory cytokines IL-1β and IL-18 [109]. The presence of the nucleotide-binding domain leucine rich repeat containing protein (NLRP3) inflammasome in platelets activated after infection by DENV has been described, inducing the production of IL-1β by platelets and platelet-derived microparticles of dengue patients [89].

3. Deregulation of the platelets' role in dengue: Hemostasis, site of virus, and immune cells

3.1. Deregulation between pro-and anticoagulant mechanisms in dengue

Hemostasis is a dynamic process in which physical and biochemical mechanisms promote blood clotting in a fast and regulated way [110]. Platelet adhesion and activation are mediated through the interactions between GP Ib-IX-V receptors with vWF and GP VI with subendothelial collagen [111]. Alternatively, when the vascular endothelium is damaged, collagen sites are exposed, facilitating platelet adhesion at these specific sites. Platelets adhere to molecules in the subendothelial tissues at the lesion site, where they aggregate and interact with leukocytes and endothelial cells, thus initiating the coagulation cascade [112]. The coagulation factors present in the bloodstream are involved in a tightly controlled activation sequence, resulting in the formation of thrombin and subsequently fibrin. These factors circulate as zymogens, which require processing by proteolysis to be activated. According to the new model of blood clotting, it occurs in three overlapping stages: initiation phase, amplification phase, and propagation phase [113].

During acute DENV infection, coagulation and fibrinolysis are activated, leading to coagulation changes and fibrinolytic parameters that may lead to disseminated intravascular coagulation (DIC) [114–116]. Funahara et al. reported that dengue patients with DIC had decreased platelet counts, transient prolongations of partial thromboplastin time (PTT) and prothrombin time (PT), and decreased levels of fibrinogen, prothrombin activity, factor VIII, antithrombin III, and plasminogen [117]. DIC leads to platelet activation, formation of fibrin, and deposition of small clots in the microcirculation, possibly contributing to organic failure. Notably, the consumption of clotting factors usually leads to paradoxical hemorrhagic disorders due to their consumption [118]. Later, it has been demonstrated that acute DIC that occurs in patients with DHF is associated with increased vascular permeability [117]. Thus, parameters such as platelet count, PTT, and PT present predictive value in the diagnosis of severe dengue [119].

The mechanisms that trigger DIC are mainly related to endothelial lesions and increased circulating TF levels [118]. Several studies have suggested that increased TF expression plays an important role in the pathogenesis of dengue. Huerta-Zepeda et al. showed that DENV regulates levels of protease-activated receptor type 1 (PAR-1) and TF in the activated endothelium [120]. These data are reinforced by the evidence of increased plasma levels of TF in dengue patients, and the expression of TF in monocytes was inversely correlated with platelet counts [121, 122]. Our previous data found that dengue patients with a good outcome showed decreased circulating levels of TF than those with a poor outcome (Severe). Similarly to TF, tissue factor pathway inhibitor (TFPI) levels were significantly lower in patients with a good outcome, but increased TFPI plasma levels were observed in severe patients. We also demonstrated that TF and TFPI levels were significantly higher among patients with hemorrhagic manifestations. In addition, DENV-1 or -2 patients were more likely to have increased levels of TF than DENV-4 patients [123]. Activation of PAR-1 is accompanied by positive regulation of adhesion molecules and production of proinflammatory cytokines [124]. The coagulation enzymes generated in DENV infection can activate PAR-1 receptors, thus increasing the increase of pro-inflammatory cytokines and leukocyte migration. These cytokines, along with coagulation enzymes (and *vice versa*), perpetuate the inflammatory response, which promotes increased interaction between activated monocytes, activated endothelial cells, and platelets. The result is a convergence of signals that lead to exacerbated expression of TF. Therefore, the coagulation and inflammation processes are closely related and establish a bidirectional relationship mediated by the activation of PARs [125].

Since hemostasis depends on the balance between coagulation and fibrinolysis, Huang et al. evaluated some coagulation parameters (platelet count and PTT) as well as fibrinolytic parameters (tPA and PAI-1) in patients with DHF and DF. Patients with DF show thrombocytopenia, PTT prolongation, and increased tPA levels, indicating coagulation activation and fibrinolysis. However, the parameters used indicated much more severe activation of coagulation and fibrinolysis in patients with DHF. In the convalescent phase, there is an increase in PAI-1 and platelet counts with concomitant decline in tPA levels and normalization of PTT, both in patients with DHF and in DF. According to the authors, the activation of coagulation and fibrinolysis during the acute phase of DENV infection is compensated by the increase of platelets and PAI-1 during the convalescence phase. These results suggest that the degree of activation of coagulation and fibrinolysis induced during dengue infection is associated with the severity of the disease [114].

3.2. Platelets as target cells for DENV replication

Platelets contain receptors related to DENV entry, such as Dendritic cell-specific intercellular adhesion molecule-3-grabbing nonintegrin (DC-SIGN) [126]. *In vitro* infection by DENV induces activation, mitochondrial dysfunction, and platelet apoptosis through mechanisms dependent on the DC-SIGN receptor [127]. A study detected DENV RNA by conventional reverse transcription polymerase chain reaction (RT-PCR) and DENV-like particles by electron microscopy in patients' platelets [128] and later confirmed the presence of viral antigen in platelets by immunofluorescence and confocal microscopy [129]. It is still unclear whether platelets are involved in the spread of viral infection. Recent data from our group have confirmed the *in vitro* interaction of DENV with platelets, leading to subsequent morphological modifications characteristic of platelet activation, such as presence of membrane extensions (filopodia), loss of cytoplasmic content and dilation of the membrane system [Azamor and Oliveira submitted]. A study using blood cells from dengue patients and rhesus monkeys experimentally infected revealed DENV antigens present in vesicles of varying sizes and often in nuclear cells like platelets. The DENV RNA was detected in a highly enriched population of rhesus platelet-characteristic CD61+ cells in the acute phase of infection, indicating that the virus may be directly linked to dysfunction and low platelet counts [130]. More recent and for the first time, authors demonstrated in fact that platelets directly bind DENV saturably and produce infectious virus. Interestingly, at 37 and 25°C, platelets replicated the positive sense single-stranded RNA genome of DENV by up to ~4-fold over 7 days, with production of viral NS1 protein. The infectivity of DENV intrinsically decayed in vitro, which was moderated by platelet-mediated generation of viable progeny. DC-SIGN and heparan sulfate proteoglycan (HSP) were implicated as coreceptors because only the combination of anti-DC-SIGN and low-molecular-weight heparin prevented binding. Thus, expression of antigen encoded by DENV is a novel consideration in the pathogen-induced thrombocytopenia mechanism [131]. Finally, very recent analyze revealed that DENV works as the primary driver of platelet activation and also enters and replicates in platelets but does not result in a productive infection of platelets. Moreover, the DENV-exposed/DENV antigen-positive platelets associate with CD14+CD16+ monocytes may mediate platelet clearance from the circulation [132].

3.3. Platelets as immune cells

Platelets, when interacting physically with leukocytes and endothelial cells, act as a kind of signaling of inflammation and immune response. When stimulated and activated, these cells initiate events, such as aggregation, formation of microparticles and exosomes [133], expression of adhesion proteins and receptors, and exocytosis of constituents present in their granules [76]. Exocytosis of α-dense granules and lysosomes releases cytokines and biological mediators with various immunological and inflammatory functions. In addition to secreting soluble mediators, platelets express receptors involved with the immune defense, such as Fc receptors that are able to recognize IgG, IgE, and IgA classes. These receptors may confer rudimentary antibacterial activities of platelets, such as the secretion of antimicrobial peptides and phagocytosis against direct interaction with bacteria, viruses, protozoa, or helminths. These immunoreceptors influence platelet adhesion activity through the modulation of integrin production [76]. Another set of receptors present on platelets with immunological action is that of TLRs. Among the 10 TLRs identified in humans, six are expressed in platelets, the TLR-1, -2, -4, -6, -8, and -9. TLR-4 has been shown to modulate sepsis and inducer of TNF-α *in vivo* [134]. TLR-2 modulates IL-1β RNA processing, inducing the production of IFN type 1 and other inflammatory cytokines [135]. The set of inflammatory, hemostatic, angiogenic, and coagulators reactions are multicellular events that include chemotaxis, adhesion, interactions between leukocytes, endothelial cells, and platelets in the walls of blood vessels. Platelets contribute to these interactions through secretion of adhesion proteins and regulation of chemokine synthesis by leukocytes and endothelial cells [136]. Molecules such as IL-1β, PAF, and P-CD62 stand out as the main mediators derived from platelets, able of activating leukocytes [137]. Studies have shown that activated platelets induce increased IL-10 expression and decreased TNF-α by monocytes [101].

Several studies have indicated that DENV infection leads to the activation of endothelial cells, which increase the expression on the surface of the E-CD62 molecule. E-CD62, as well as P-CD62, are adhesion molecules responsible for platelet adhesion to endothelial cells [113, 138]. In addition to the endothelium, P-CD62 is expressed on the surface of activated platelets, promoting their interaction with leukocytes and formation of aggregates between platelets and monocytes and/ or neutrophils in primates [139]. Platelet-monocyte aggregates are also observed in DENV-infected patients, leading to the synthesis of IL-1β, CXCL8/ IL-8, CCL4/ MCP-1, and IL-10 by monocytes [107]. The formation of cell aggregates results in an increase in the inflammatory response in dengue, as well as contributing to the generation of thrombocytopenia both by the physical retention of cells, by lowering the number of circulating cells and by the induction of cell death [140]. In 1992, Butthep et al. showed that platelets, as well as neutrophils and lymphocytes, preferentially bind to endothelial cells exposed to DENV, compared to cells not exposed to DENV. It has been suggested that increased platelet endothelial cell binding may contribute to thrombocytopenia in dengue patients [141]. Protein disulfide isomerase (PDI), an endoplasmic reticular protein, is located on the surface of platelets [142] and is involved in the regulation of integrin-mediated platelet aggregation, since anti-PDI antibodies block platelet adhesion and aggregation [143]. Previous studies have demonstrated that platelet surface PDI can be recognized by anti-NS1 antibodies. Rachman and co-workers observed a similar kinetic profile between anti-NS1 and PDI antibodies [144]. PDI enzyme activity and platelet aggregation were reduced with anti-NS1 action. Amino acid residues 311–330 (P311–330) of NS1 represent an epitope that shares sequence homology with the PDI thiorretoxin domain [145]. In contrast, although the serum of dengue patients inhibits platelet aggregation, there is no correlation between anti-NS1 and PDI with platelet aggregation dysfunction, suggesting that other mechanisms may be involved in the inhibition of platelet aggregation [144, 145]. Platelets are responsible for the maintenance of vascular integrity due to the constitutive release of pro-angiogenic cytokines and growth factors. The α-granule-derived molecules such as angiopoietin-1, α and β-catenins, and PAF bind to specific receptors on the surface of endothelial cells, causing intracellular signaling that stabilizes the intercellular adhesion junctions [146]. Angiopoietins, key molecules of vascular integrity, are also stored in platelets. Both dengue-associated thrombocytopenia and endothelial activation are associated with an imbalance in the ratio of angiopoietin-2: angiopoietin-1 plasmatic. Studies have shown that there is an inverse correlation between angiopoietin-1 and plasma extravasation markers but a direct correlation between angiopoietin-2 and markers of plasma extravasation in patients with DHF/DSS [147]. Hottz et al. demonstrated that DENV-infected patients who showed signs of increased vascular permeability demonstrated a higher percentage of platelets and platelet-derived microparticles (MP) expressing IL-1β and caspase-1 activator compared to patients who had no evidence change in vascular permeability. These results were confirmed in experiments in which platelet-derived MPs exposed to DENV caused an increase in the permeability of endothelial cells that was blocked by IL-1Ra [127].

More recently, proteome analysis related to platelet activating signaling from platelets from dengue patients demonstrated an increase of PAR-4 (F2RL3), G protein subunits (GNA12 and GNA14), and p38 MAPK (MAPK14), in which potentially contributing to increased platelet activation during dengue infection. Moreover, dengue patients had increased P-CD62 surface expression on platelets from patients presenting dengue with warning signs and severe dengue syndromes compared to mild dengue. In agreement, they observed exhaustion of the granule-stored chemokine PF4/CXCL4 in platelets from patients with dengue [148], similarly to another study reported that patients with severe dengue have lower levels of PF4/CXCL4 in plasma when compared to mild dengue patients [149].

4. Conclusion

Platelets are cellular fragments derived from hematopoietic precursors megakaryocytes, primarily associated with coagulation and hemostasis and also with inflammation, immune response, angiogenesis, and extracellular matrix synthesis. In fact, platelets contain several preformed molecules, large amounts of mRNA, and the packaged translational process required to synthesize new biologically active proteins, including growth factors, cytokines, and chemokines. Platelets are one of the major cell populations affected in dengue, once both thrombocytopenia and platelet dysfunction are common manifestations of infection and strongly related to the patient's clinical outcome. Dysfunction of platelets is implicated in prothrombotic complications associated with severe cases of dengue. Thus, platelets could be considered cells that are active against the anti-DENV immune response, and therefore, thrombocytopenia is a key prognostic factor in the immunopathogenesis of dengue.

Abbreviations

DENV	dengue virus
E	envelope
M	membrane
C	capsid
prM	pre-Membrane
NS	nonstructural

DF	dengue fever or dengue fever without signs of alarm
DHF	dengue hemorrhagic fever
DSS	dengue shock syndrome
WHO	World Health Organization
DFwWS	dengue fever with warning signals
ADE	antibody-dependent infection
IFNs	interferons
NKs	natural killer cells
pDC	plasmacytoid dendritic cells
DCs	dendritic cells
IFN-α/β	type I IFNs
IFN-γ	or IFN-type II
HLA	human leukocyte antigen
APCs	antigen-presenting cells
ICAM-1	intracellular adhesion molecule-1
VCAM-1	vascular cell adhesion molecule-1
E-CD62	E-selectin
TGF-β	transforming growth factor-beta-receptor
sST2	soluble IL-1 receptor type 1 protein
sTRAIL	tumor necrosis factor-related apoptosis-inducing ligand
PT	profound thrombocytopenia
TPO	thrombopoietin
DENV-EIII	DENV-envelope protein domain III
P-CD62	P-selectin
PAF	platelet-activating factor
vWF	von Willebrand factor
ADP	adenosine diphosphate
TXA_2	thromboxane A_2
GP	glycoprotein
RGD sequence	Arginine-Glycine-Asparagine peptide sequence

TF	tissue factor
βTG	beta thromboglobulin
PF4/CXCL4	platelet factor 4
PGD2	Prostaglandin D2
TLRs	toll-like receptors
NLRP3	nucleotide-binding domain leucine rich repeat containing protein
DIC	disseminated intravascular coagulation
PTT	partial thromboplastin time
PT	prothrombin time
PAR-1	protease-activated receptor type 1
TFPI	tissue factor pathway inhibitor
DC-SIGN	dendritic cell-specific intercellular adhesion molecule-3-grabbing nonintegrin
RT-PCR	reverse transcription polymerase chain reaction
HSP	heparan sulfate proteoglycan
PDI	protein disulfide isomerase
MP	microparticles

Author details

Tamiris Azamor da Costa Barros[1,2] and Luzia Maria de-Oliveira-Pinto[1]*

*Address all correspondence to: lpinto@ioc.fiocruz.br

1 Laboratory of Viral Immunology, Instituto Oswaldo Cruz, Fiocruz, Rio de Janeiro, Brazil

2 Laboratory of Immunological Technology, Instituto de Tecnologia em Imunobiológicos Bio-Manguinhos, Fiocruz, Rio de Janeiro, Brazil

References

[1] WHO and the Special Programme for Research and Training in Tropical Diseases (TDR). Dengue guidelines for diagnosis, treatment, prevention and control: new edition. http://www.who.int/rpc/guidelines/9789241547871/en/. (2009, accessed13 February 2017)

[2] Lindenbach BD, Rice CM. Mint: Flaviviridae: the viruses and their replication. In Knipe KM, Howley PM, editors. Fieds Virology. 2001. Philadelphia, PA: Lippicott-Wlikins, pp.991-1041

[3] Kuhn RJ, Zang W, Rossman MG, Pletnev SV, Cover J, Lenches E, Jones CT, Mukhopadhuay S, Chipman PR, Strauss EG, Baker TS, Stauss JH. Mint: Structure of dengue virus: Implications for flavivirus organization, mutation and fusion. Cell. 2002;**108**(5):717-725

[4] Chambers TJ, Hahn CS, Galler R, Rice CM. Mint: Flavivirus genome organization, expression and replication. Annual Review of Microbiology. 1990;**44**:649-688

[5] Mukhopadhyay S, Kuhn RJ, Rossmann MG. Mint: A structural perspective of the flavivirus life cycle. Nature Reviews Microbiology. 2005;**3**(1):13-22

[6] Qi RF, Zhang L, Chi CW. Mint: Biological characteristics of dengue virus and potential targets for drug design. Acta Biochimica et Biophysica Sinica. 2008;**40**(2):91-101

[7] Gubler DJ. Mint: Epidemic dengue/dengue hemorrhagic fever as a public health, social and economic problem in the 21st century. Trends in Microbiology. 2002;**10**(2):100-103

[8] Bäck AT, Lundkvist Å. Mint: Dengue viruses–an overview. Infection Ecology & Epidemiology. 2013;**3**:19839

[9] Simmons CP, Farrar JJ, van Vinh Chau N, Wills B. Mint: Dengue. New England Journal of Medicine. 2012;**366**(15):1423-1432

[10] Barniol J, Gaczkowski R, Barbato EV, da Cunha RV, Salgado D, Martínez E, Jaenisch T. Mint: Usefulness and applicability of the revised dengue case classification by disease: Multi-centre study in 18 countries. BMC infectious diseases. 2011;**11**(1):106

[11] Halstead SB, Nimmannitya S, Cohe SN. Mint: Observations related to pathogenesis of dengue hemorrhagic fever. IV. Relation of disease severity to antibody response and virus recovered. The Yale Journal of Biology and Medicine. 1970;**42**:311-328

[12] Halstead SB, Porterfield JS, O'Rourke EJ. Mint: Enhancement of dengue virus infection in monocytes by flavivirus antisera. The American Journal of Tropical Medicine and Hygiene. 1980;**29**:638-642

[13] Mongkolsapaya J, Dejnirattisai W, Xu X, et al. Mint: Original antigenic sin and apoptosis in the pathogenesis of dengue hemorrhagic fever. Nature Medicine. 2003;**9**:921-927

[14] Rothman AL. Mint: Immunity to dengue virus: A tale of original antigenic sin and tropical cytokine storms. Nature Reviews Immunology. 2011;**11**(8):532-543

[15] Valdés K, Alvarez M, Pupo M, Vázquez S, Rodríguez R, Guzmán MG. Mint: Human dengue antibodies against structural and nonstructural proteins. Clinical and diagnostic laboratory immunology. 2000;**7**(5):856-857

[16] Churdboonchart V, Bhamarapravati N, Peampramprecha S, Sirinavin S. Mint: Antibodies against dengue viral proteins in primary and secondary dengue hemorrhagic fever. The American Journal of Tropical Medicine and Hygiene. 1991;**44**(5):481-493

[17] Rothman AL. Mint: Dengue: Defining protective versus pathologic immunity. Journal of Clinical Investigation. 2004;**113**(7):946-951

[18] Nybakken GE, Oliphant T, Johnson S, Burke S, Diamond MS, Fremont DH. Mint: Structural basis of West Nile virus neutralization by a therapeutic antibody. Nature 2005;**437**(7059):764-769

[19] Vogt MR, Moesker B, Goudsmit J, Jongeneelen M, Austin SK, Oliphant T, et al. Mint: Human monoclonal antibodies against West Nile virus induced by natural infection neutralize at a postattachment step. Journal of Virology. 2009;**83**(13):6494-6507

[20] Halstead SB. Mint: Neutralization and antibody-dependent enhancement of dengue viruses. Advances in Virus Research 2003;**60**:421-467

[21] Rivino L. Mint: T cell immunity to dengue virus and implications for vaccine design. Expert Review of Vaccines. 2016;**15**:443-453

[22] Simmons CP, Dong T, Chau NV, et al. Mint: Early T-cell responses to dengue virus epitopes in Vietnamese adults with secondary dengue virus infections. Journal of Virology. 2005;**79**:5665-5675

[23] Rivino L, Tan AT, Chia A, et al. Mint: Defining CD8+ T cell determinants during human viral infection in populations of Asian ethnicity. Journal of Immunology Baltim Md. 2013;**191**:4010-4019

[24] Malavige GN, Ogg G. Mint: Pathogenesis of severe dengue infection. Ceylon Medical Journal. 2012;**57**(3):97-100

[25] Samuel CE. Mint: Antiviral actions of interferons. Clinical Microbiology Reviews. 2001; **14**(4):778-809

[26] Le Bon A, Tough DF. Mint: Links between innate and adaptive immunity via type I interferon. Current Opinion in Immunology. 2002;**14**(4):432-436

[27] Jones M, Davidson A, Hibbert L, Gruenwald P, Schlaak J, Ball S, Jacobs M. Mint: Dengue virus inhibits alpha interferon signaling by reducing STAT2 expression. Journal of Virology. 2005;**79**(9):5414-5420

[28] Ashour J, Laurent-Rolle M., Shi PY, García-Sastre A. Mint: NS5 of dengue virus mediates STAT2 binding and degradation. Journal of Virology. 2009;**83**(11):5408-5418

[29] Muñoz-Jordán JL1, Laurent-Rolle M, Ashour J, Martínez-Sobrido L, Ashok M, Lipkin WI, García-Sastre A. Mint: Inhibition of alpha/beta interferon signaling by the NS4B protein of flaviviruses. Journal of Virology. 2005;**79**(13):8004-8013

[30] Gandini M, Gras C, Azeredo EL, de Oliveira Pinto LM., Smith N, Despres P, Herbeuval JP. Mint: Dengue virus activates membrane TRAIL relocalization and IFN-α production by human plasmacytoid dendritic cells *In vitro* and *In vivo*. PLoS Neglected Tropical Diseases. 2013;**7**(6):e2257

[31] Commins SP, Borish L, Steinke JW. Mint: Immunologic messenger molecules: Cytokines, interferons, and chemokines. Journal of Allergy and Clinical Immunology. 2010;**125**(2): S53-S72

[32] Kurane I, Innis BL, Nimmannitya S, Nisalak A, Meager A, Janus J, Ennis FA. Mint: Activation of T lymphocytes in dengue virus infections. High levels of soluble interleukin 2 receptor, soluble CD4, soluble CD8, interleukin 2, and interferon-gamma in sera of children with dengue. Journal of Clinical Investigation. 1991;**88**(5):1473

[33] Dewi BE, Takasaki T, Kurane I. Mint: In vitro assessment of human endothelial cell permeability: Effects of inflammatory cytokines and dengue virus infection. Journal of Virological Methods. 2004;**121**(2):171-180

[34] Azeredo EL, Zagne SM, Santiago MA, Gouvea AS, Santana AA, Neves-Souza PC, Kubelka CF. Mint: Characterisation of lymphocyte response and cytokine patterns in patients with dengue fever. Immunobiology. 2001;**204**(4):494-507

[35] Bozza FA, Cruz OG, Zagne SM, Azeredo EL, Nogueira RM, Assis EF, Kubelka CF. Mint: Multiplex cytokine profile from dengue patients: MIP-1beta and IFN-gamma as predictive factors for severity. BMC Infectious Diseases. 2008;**8**(1):86

[36] Juffrie M, Meer GV, Hack CE, Haasnoot K, Veerman AJ, Thijs LG. Mint: Inflammatory mediators in dengue virus infection in children: Interleukin-6 and its relation to C-reactive protein and secretory phospholipase A2. The American Journal of Tropical Medicine and Hygiene. 2001;**65**(1):70-75

[37] Mustafa AS, Elbishbishi EA, Agarwal R, Chaturvedi UC. Mint: Elevated levels of interleukin-13 and IL-18 in patients with dengue hemorrhagic fever. FEMS Immunology & Medical Microbiology. 2001;**30**(3):229-233

[38] Nguyen TH, Lei HY, Nguyen TL, Lin YS, Huang KJ, Le BL, Lin CF, Yeh TM, Do QH, Vu TQ, Chen LC, Huang JH, Lam TM, Liu CC, Halstead SB. Mint: Dengue hemorrhagic fever in infants: a study of clinical and cytokine profiles. The Journal of Infectious Diseases. 2004;**189**(2):221-232

[39] Raghupathy R, Chaturvedi UC, Al-Sayer H, Elbishbishi EA, Agarwal R, Nagar R, Kapoor S, Misra A, Mathur A, Nusrat H, Azizieh F, Khan MA, Mustafa AS. Mint: Elevated levels of IL-8 in dengue hemorrhagic fever. Journal of medical virology. 1998;**56**(3):280-285

[40] Restrepo BN, Isaza DM, Salazar CL, Ramírez R, Ospina M, Alvarez LG. Mint: Serum levels of interleukin-6, tumor necrosis factor-alpha and interferon-gama in infants with and without dengue. Revista da Sociedade Brasileira de Medicina Tropical. 2008;**41**(1):6-10

[41] Chaturvedi UC, Agarwal R, Elbishbishi EA, Mustafa AS. Mint: Cytokine cascade in dengue hemorrhagic fever: Implications for pathogenesis. FEMS Immunology & Medical Microbiology. 2000;**28**(3):183-188

[42] Miller JL, M deWet BJ, Martinez-Pomares L, Radcliffe CM, Dwek RA, Rudd PM, Gordon S. Mint: The mannose receptor mediates dengue virus infection of macrophages. PLoS Pathogens. 2008;**4**(2):e17

[43] Libraty DH, Endy TP, Houng HSH, Green S, Kalayanarooj S, Suntayakorn S, Rothman AL. Mint: Differing influences of virus burden and immune activation on disease severity in secondary dengue-3 virus infections. Journal of Infectious Diseases. 2002;**185**(9): 1213-1221

[44] Arias J, Valero N, Mosquera J, Montiel M, Reyes E, Larreal Y, Alvarez-Mon M. Mint: Increased expression of cytokines, soluble cytokine receptors, soluble apoptosis ligand and apoptosis in dengue. Virology 2014;**452**:42-51

[45] Basu A, Jain P, Gangodkar SV, Shetty S, Ghosh K. Mint: Dengue 2 virus inhibits *in vitro* megakaryocytic colony formation and induces apoptosis in thrombopoietin-inducible megakaryocytic differentiation from cord blood CD34+ cells. FEMS Immunology & Medical Microbiology. 2008;**53**:46-51

[46] Nakao S, Lai C-J, Young NS. Mint: Dengue virus, a flavivirus, propagates in human bone marrow progenitors and hematopoietic cell lines. Blood. 1989;**74**:1235-1240

[47] Azeredo EL de, Monteiro RQ, De-Oliveira pinto LM. Mint: Thrombocytopenia in dengue: Interrelationship between virus and the imbalance between coagulation and fibrinolysis and inflammatory mediators. Mediators of Inflammation. 2015;**3**:138-142

[48] WHO. WHO Recommended Surveillance Standards. Second edition. Global Alert and Respose - Disease Outbreak Reported. 2002. 116

[49] Jayashree K, Manasa GC, Pallavi P, Manjunath GV. Mint: Evaluation of platelets as predictive parameters in dengue fever. Indian Journal of Hematology and Blood Transfusion. 2011;**27**(3):127-130

[50] Mitrakul C. Mint: Bleeding problem in dengue haemorrhagic fever: Platelets and coagulation changes. Southeast Asian Journal of Tropical Medicine and Public Health. 1987;**18**(3): 407-412

[51] Srichaikul T, Nimmannitya S. Mint: Haematology in dengue and dengue haemorrhagic fever. Best Practice & Research Clinical Haematology. 2000;**13**(2):261-276

[52] Dhanoa A, Rajasekaram G, Hassan SS, Ramadas A, Azreen Adnan NA, Lau CF, Chan TS, Ngim CF. Mint: Risk factors and clinical outcome of profound thrombocytopenia in adult patients with DENV infections. Platelets. 2017;**28**(7):724-727

[53] Chaudhary R, Khetan D, Sinha S, Sinha P, Sonker A, Pandey P, Das SS, Agarwal P, Ray V. Mint: Transfusion support to dengue patients in a hospital based blood transfusion service in north India. Transfusion and Apheresis Science. 2006;**35**(3):239-244

[54] Makroo RN, Raina V, Kumar P, Kanth RK. Mint: Role of platelet transfusion in the management of dengue patients in a tertiary care hospital. Asian Journal of Transfusion Science. 2007;**1**(1):4

[55] Khan Assir MZ, Kamran U, Ahmad HI, Bashir S, Mansoor H, Anees SB, Akram J. Mint: Effectiveness of platelet transfusion in dengue Fever: a randomized controlled trial. Transfus Med Hemother. 2013;**40**(5):362-368

[56] Hottz E, Tolley ND, Zimmerman GA, Weyrich AS, Bozza FA. Mint: Platelets in dengue infection. Drug Discovery Today: Disease Mechanisms. 2011;**8**(1):e33-e38

[57] Kho LK, Wulur H, Himawan T. Mint: Blood and bone marrow changes in dengue haemorrhagic fever. Paediatrica Indonesiana. 1972;**12**(1):31

[58] La Russa VF, Innis BL. Mint: Mechanisms of dengue virus-induced bone marrow suppression. Baillière's Clinical Haematology. 1995;**8**(1):249-270

[59] Klinger MH, Jelkmann W. Mint: Review: Role of blood platelets in infection and inflammation. Journal of Interferon & Cytokine Research. 2002;**22**(9):913-922

[60] Badalucco S, Di Buduo CA, Campanelli R, Pallotta I, Catarsi P, Rosti V, Kaplan DL, Barosi G, Massa M, Balduini A. Mint: Involvement of TGFβ1 in autocrine regulation of proplatelet formation in healthy subjects and patients with primary myelofibrosis. Haematologica and Haematology. 2013

[61] de Sauvage FJ1, Hass PE, Spencer SD, Malloy BE, Gurney AL, Spencer SA, Darbonne WC, Henzel WJ, Wong SC, Kuang WJ, et al. Mint: Stimulation of megakaryocytopoiesis and thrombopoiesis by the c-Mpl ligand. Nature. 1994;**369**(6481):533-538

[62] Gurney AL, Carver-Moore K, de Sauvage F, Moore MW. Mint: Thrombocytopenia in c-mpl-deficient mice. Science. 1994;**265**(5177):1445-1447

[63] Putintseva E, Vega G, Fernandez L. Mint: Alterations in thrombopoiesis in patients with thrombocytopenia produced by dengue hemorrhagic fever. Nouvelle Revue Francaise D'Hematologie. 1985;**28**(5):269-273

[64] Matondang AV, Widodo D, Zulkarnain I, Rengganis I, Trihandini I, Inada K, Endo S. Mint: The correlation between thrombopoietin and platelet count in adult dengue viral infection patients. Acta Medica Indonesiana. 2004;**36**(2):62-69

[65] Lin GL, Chang HH, Lien TS, Chen PK, Chan H, Su MT, Liao CY, Sun DS. Mint: Suppressive effect of dengue virus envelope protein domain III on megakaryopoiesis. Virulence. 2017;**8**(8):1719-1731

[66] Wang S, He R, Patarapotikul J, Innis BL, AR. Mint: Antibody-enhanced binding of dengue-2 virus to human platelets. Virology. 1995;**213**(1):254-257

[67] Huang KJ, Li SY, Chen SC, Liu HS, Lin YS, Yeh TM, Liu CC, Lei HY. Mint: Manifestation of thrombocytopenia in dengue-2-virus-infected mice. The Journal of General Virology. 2000;**81**(Pt 9):2177-2182

[68] Falconar AK. Mint: The dengue virus nonstructural-1 protein (NS1) generates antibodies to common epitopes on human blood clotting, integrin/adhesin proteins and binds to human endothelial cells: Potential implications in haemorrhagic fever pathogenesis. Archives of Virology. 1997;**142**(5):897-916

[69] Ojha A, Nandi D, Batra H, Singhal R, Annarapu GK, Bhattacharyya S, Seth T, Dar L, Medigeshi GR, Vrati S, Vikram NK, Guchhait P. Platelet activation determines the severity of thrombocytopenia in dengue infection. Scientific Reports. 2017;**7**:41697

[70] Wan SW, Lin CF, Yeh TM, Liu CC, Liu HS, Wang S, Ling P, Anderson R, Lei HY, Lin YS. Mint: Autoimmunity in dengue pathogenesis. Journal of the Formosan Medical Association. 2013;**112**(1):3-11

[71] Lin CF, Lei HY, Liu CC, Liu HS, Yeh TM, Wang ST, Yang TI, Sheu FC, Kuo CF, Lin YS. Mint: Generation of IgM anti-platelet autoantibody in dengue patients. Journal of Medical Virology. 2001;**63**(2):143-149

[72] Lin CF, Lei HY, Shiau AL, Liu CC, Liu HS, Yeh TM, Chen SH, Lin YS. Mint: Antibodies from dengue patient sera cross-react with endothelial cells and induce damage. Journal of Medical Virology. 2003;**69**(1):82-90

[73] Lin YS, Yeh TM, Lin CF, Wan SW, Chuang YC, Hsu TK, Liu HS, Liu CC, Anderson R, Lei HY. Mint: Molecular mimicry between virus and host and its implications for dengue disease pathogenesis. Experimental Biology and Medicine. 2011;**236**(5):515-523

[74] Chen M, Geng JG. Mint: P-selectin mediates adhesion of leukocytes, platelets, and cancer cells in inflammation, thrombosis, and cancer growth and metastasis. Archivum Immunologiae et Therapiae Experimentalis. 2006;**54**(2):75-84

[75] Souza DG, Fagundes CT, Sousa LP, Amaral FA, Souza RS, Souza AL, Kroon EG, Sachs D, Cunha FQ, Bukin E, Atrasheuskaya A, Ignatyev G, Teixeira MM. Mint: Essential role of platelet activating factor receptor in the pathogenesis of dengue virus infection. PNAS. 2009;**106**(33):14138-14143

[76] Basuki PS. Mint: A glance at the von Willebrand factor in dengue virus infection. Southeast Asian J Trop Med Public Health. 2003;**34**(3):559-563

[77] Alonzo MT, Lacuesta TL, Dimaano EM, Kurosu T, Suarez LA, Mapua CA, Akeda Y, Matias RR, Kuter DJ, Nagata S, Natividad FF, Oishi K. Mint: Platelet apoptosis and apoptotic platelet clearance by macrophages in secondary dengue virus infections. Journal of Infectious Diseases. 2012;**205**(8):1321-1329

[78] Hottz ED, Lopes JF, Freitas C, Valls-de-Souza R, Oliveira MF, Bozza MT, Bozza PT. Mint: Platelets mediate increased endothelium permeability in dengue through NLRP3-inflammasome activation. Blood. 2013;**122**(20):3405-3414

[79] Cimmino G, Golino P. Mint: Platelet biology and receptor pathways. Journal of Cardiovascular Translational Research. 2013;**6**(3):299-309

[80] Torre D, Pugliese A. Mint: Platelets and HIV-1 infection: Old and new aspects. Current HIV Research. 2008;**6**:411-418

[81] Michelson AD, MacGregor H, Barnard MR, Kestin AS, Rohrer MJ, Valeri CR. Mint: Reversible inhibition of human platelet activation by hypothermia in vivo and in vitro. Thrombosis and Haemostasis. 1994;**71**(5):633-640

[82] Davì G, Ciabattoni G, Consoli A, Mezzetti A, Falco A, Santarone S, Patrono C. Mint: In vivo formation of 8-Iso-prostaglandin F2α and platelet activation in diabetes mellitus effects of improved metabolic control and vitamin E supplementation. Circulation. 1999;**99**(2):224-229

[83] Davì G, Patrono C. Mint: Platelet activation and atherothrombosis. New England Journal of Medicine. 2007;**357**(24):2482-2494

[84] Jennings LK. Mint: Mechanisms of platelet activation: Need for new strategies to protect against platelet-mediated atherothrombosis. Thrombosis and Haemostasis. 2009;**102**(2):248-257

[85] Vieira-de-Abreu A, Campbell RA, Weyrich AS, Zimmerman GA. Platelets: Versatile effector cells in hemostasis, inflammation, and the immune continuum. Seminars in Immunopathology. 2012;**34**:5-30

[86] Jurk K, Kehrel BE. Mint: Platelets: physiology and biochemistry. Semin Thromb Hemost. 2005;**31**(4):381-92

[87] Calvete JJ, Henschen A, González-Rodríguez J. Mint: Assignment of disulphide bonds in human platelet GPIIIa. A disulphide pattern for the beta-subunits of the integrin family. The Biochemical Journal. 1991;**274**:63-71

[88] Weyrich AS, Elstad MR, McEver RP, McIntyre TM, Moore KL, Morrissey JH, Prescott SM, Zimmerman GA. Mint: Activated platelets signal chemokine synthesis by human monocytes. The Journal of Clinical Investigation. 1996;**97**:1525-1534

[89] Hottz ED, Medeiros-de-Moraes IM, Vieira-de-Abreu A, de Assis EF, Vals-de-Souza R, Castro-Faria-Neto HC, Weyrich AS, Zimmerman GA, Bozza FA, Bozza PT. Mint: Platelet activation and apoptosis modulate monocyte inflammatory responses in dengue. Journal of Immunology 2014;**193**:1864-1872

[90] Larsen E, Celi U, Gilbert GE, Furie BC, Erban JK, Bonfanti R, Wagner DD, Furie B. Mint: PADGEM protein: a receptor that mediates the interaction of activated platelets with neutrophils and monocytes. Cell. 1989;**59**:305-312

[91] Tsai JJ, Jen YH, Chang JS, Hsiao HM, Noisakran S, Perng GC. Mint: Frequency alterations in key innate immune cell components in the peripheral blood of dengue patients detected by FACS analysis. Journal of Innate Immunity. 2011;**3**:530-540

[92] Ghosh K, Gangodkar S, Jain P, Shetty S, Ramjee S, Poddar P, Basu A. Mint: Imaging the interaction between dengue 2 virus and human blood platelets using atomic force and electron microscopy. Journal of electron microscopy. 2008;**57**(3):113-118

[93] Shi G, Morrell CN. Mint: Platelets as initiators and mediators of inflammation at the vessel wall. Thrombosis research. 2011;**127**(5):387-390

[94] Rondina MT, Schwertz H, Harris ES, Kraemer BF, Campbell RA, Mackman N, Grissom CK, Weyrich AS, Zimmerman GA. Mint: The septic milieu triggers expression of spliced tissue factor mRNA in human platelets. Journal of Thrombosis and Haemostasis. 2011;**9**(4): 748-58

[95] Zimmerman GA, Weyrich AS. Mint: Signal-dependent protein synthesis by activated platelets new pathways to altered phenotype and function. Arteriosclerosis, thrombosis, and vascular biology. 2008;**28**(3):s17-s24

[96] Weyrich AS, Schwertz H, Kraiss LW, Zimmerman GA. Mint: Protein synthesis by platelets: historical and new perspectives. Journal of Thrombosis and Haemostasis. 2009;**7**(2):241-246

[97] Brass LF. Mint: Thrombin and platelet activation. Chest. 2003;**124**:18S-25S

[98] Davi G, Patrono C. Mint: Platelet activation and atherothrombosis. The New England Journal of Medicine. 2007;**357**:2482-2494

[99] Offermanns S. Mint: Activation of platelet function through G protein-coupled receptors. Circulation Research. 2006;**99**:1293-1304

[100] Li Z, Delaney MK, O'Brien KA, Du X. Mint: Signaling during platelet adhesion and activation. Arteriosclerosis, Thrombosis, and Vascular Biology. 2010;**30**:2341-2349

[101] Srichaikul T, Nimmannitya S, Sripaisarn T, Kamolsilpa M, Pulgate C. Mint: Platelet function during the acute phase of dengue hemorrhagic fever. The Southeast Asian Journal of Tropical Medicine and Public Health. 1989;**20**(1):19-25

[102] Yang KD, Lee CS, Hwang KP, Chu ML, Shaio MF. Mint: A model to study cytokine profiles in primary and heterologously secondary Dengue-2 virus infections. Acta virologica. 1995;**39**(1):19-21

[103] Preeyasombat C, Treepongkaruna S, Sriphrapradang A, Choubtum L. Mint: The role of prostacyclin (PGI2) and thromboxane A2 (TXA2) in pathogenesis of dengue hemorrhagic fever (DHF). Journal of the Medical Association of Thailand. 1999;**82**:S16-S21

[104] Gudbrandsdottir S, Hasselbalch HC, Nielsen CH. Mint: Activated platelets enhance IL-10 secretion and reduce TNF-α secretion by monocytes. The Journal of Immunology. 2013;**191**(8):4059-4067

[105] Assoian RK, Komoriya A, Meyers CA, Miller DM, Sporn MB. Mint: Transforming growth factor-beta in human platelets. Identification of a major storage site, purification, and characterization. Journal of Biological Chemistry. 1983;**258**(11):7155-7160

[106] Djamiatun K, Faradz SM, Setiati TE, Netea MG, van der Ven AJ, Dolmans WM. Mint: Increase of plasminogen activator inhibitor-1 and decrease of transforming growth factor-B1 in children with dengue haemorrhagic fever in Indonesia. Journal of Tropical Pediatrics. 2011

[107] Andersson PO, Olsson A, Wadenvik H. Mint: Reduced transforming growth factor-β1 production by mononuclear cells from patients with active chronic idiopathic thrombocytopenic purpura. British Journal of Haematology. 2002;**116**(4):862-867

[108] Janeway Jr CA, Medzhitov R. Mint: Innate immune recognition. Annual Review of Immunology. 2002;**20**(1):197-216

[109] Place DE, Kanneganti TD. Mint: Recent advances in inflammasome biology. Current Opinion in Immunology. 2017;**50**:32-38

[110] Qu Z, Chaikof EL. Mint: Interface between hemostasis and adaptive immunity. Current Opinion in Immunology. 2010;**22**(5):634-642

[111] Rumbaut RE, Thiagarajan P. Mint: Platelet-vessel wall interactions in hemostasis and thrombosis. Synthesis Lectures on Integrated Systems Physiology: From Molecule to Function. 2010;**2**(1):1-75

[112] Furie B, Furie BC. Mint: Mechanisms of thrombus formation. New England Journal of Medicine. 2008;**359**(9):938-949

[113] Hoffman M. Mint: A cell-based model of coagulation and the role of factor VIIa. Blood Reviews. 2003;**17**:S1-S5

[114] Huang YH, Liu CC, Wang ST, Lei HY, Liu HS, Lin YS, Yeh TM. Mint: Activation of coagulation and fibrinolysis during dengue virus infection. Journal of medical virology. 2001;**63**(3):247-251

[115] Sosothikul D, Seksarn P, Pongsewalak S, Thisyakorn U, Lusher J. Mint: Activation of endothelial cells, coagulation and fibrinolysis in children with dengue virus infection. Thrombosis and Haemostasis. 2007;**97**(4):627-634

[116] Wills B, Tran VN, Nguyen TH, Truong TT, Tran TN, Nguyen MD, Tran VD, Nguyen VV, Dinh TT, Farrar J. Mint: Hemostatic changes in Vietnamese children with mild dengue correlate with the severity of vascular leakage rather than bleeding. The American Journal of Tropical Medicine and Hygiene. 2009;**81**(4):638-644

[117] Funahara Y, Sumarmo, Shirahata A, Setiabudy-Dharma R. Mint: DHF characterized by acute type DIC with increased vascular permeability. The Southeast Asian Journal of Tropical Medicine and Public Health 1987;**18**(3):346-350

[118] Bick RL. Mint: Disseminated intravascular coagulation: A review of etiology, pathophysiology, diagnosis, and management: Guidelines for care. Official Journal of the International Academy of Clinical and Applied Thrombosis/Hemostasis. 2002;**8**(1):1-31

[119] Liu JW, Lee IK, Wang L, Chen RF, Yang KD. The usefulness of clinical-practice-based laboratory data in facilitating the diagnosis of dengue illness. BioMed Research International. 2013;**2013**:198797

[120] Huerta-Zepeda A, Cabello-Gutiérrez C, Cime-Castillo J, Monroy-Martínez V, Manjarrez-Zavala ME, Gutiérrez-Rodríguez M, Izaguirre R, Ruiz-Ordaz BH. Mint: Crosstalk between coagulation and inflammation during dengue virus infection. Thombosis and Haemostasis-Stuttgart. 2008;**99**(5):936

[121] Wills BA, Oragui EE, Stephens AC, Daramola OA, Dung NM, Loan HT, Chau NV, Chambers M, Stepniewska K, Farrar JJ, Levin M. Mint: Coagulation abnormalities in dengue hemorrhagic fever: serial investigations in 167 Vietnamese children with dengue shock syndrome. Clinical infectious diseases. 2002;**35**(3):277-285

[122] de Azeredo EL, Kubelka CF, Alburquerque LM, Barbosa LS, Damasco PV, Avila CA, Motta-Castro AR, da Cunha RV, Monteiro RQ. Tissue factor expression on monocytes from patients with severe dengue fever. Blood Cells, Molecules & Diseases. 2010;**45**(4):334-335

[123] Leal de Azeredo E, Solórzano VE, de Oliveira DB, Marinho CF, de Souza LJ, da Cunha RV, Damasco PV, Kubelka CF, de-Oliveira-Pinto LM. Mint: Increased circulating procoagulant and anticoagulant factors as TF and TFPI according to severity or infecting serotypes in human dengue infection. Microbes and Infection. 2017;**19**(1):62-68

[124] Levi M, van der Poll T, Büller HR. Mint: Bidirectional relation between inflammation and coagulation. Circulation. 2004;**109**(22):2698-2704

[125] Ruf W. Mint: Protease-activated receptor signaling in the regulation of inflammation. Critical Care Medicine. 2004;**32**(5):S287-S292

[126] Boukour S, Massé JM, Bénit L, Dubart-Kupperschmitt A, Cramer EM. Mint: Lentivirus degradation and DC-SIGN expression by human platelets and megakaryocytes. Journal of Thrombosis and Haemostasis. 2006;**4**(2):426-435

[127] Hottz ED, Oliveira MF, Nunes PC, Nogueira RMR, Valls-de-Souza R, Da Poian AT, Mint BFA. Dengue induces platelet activation, mitochondrial dysfunction and cell death through mechanisms that involve DC-SIGN and caspases. Journal of Thrombosis and Haemostasis. 2013;**11**(5):951-962

[128] Noisakran S, Gibbons RV, Songprakhon P, Jairungsri A, Ajariyakhajorn C, Nisalak A, Jarman RG, Malasit P, Chokephaibulkit K, Perng GC. Mint: Detection of dengue virus in platelets isolated from dengue patients. The Southeast Asian Journal of Tropical Medicine and Public Health. 2009;**40**(2):253-262

[129] Noisakran S, Chokephaibulkit K, Songprakhon P, Onlamoon N, Hsiao HM, Villinger F, Perng GC. Mint: A re-evaluation of the mechanisms leading to dengue Hemorrhagic fever. Annals of the New York Academy of Sciences. 2009;**1171**(s1):E24-E35

[130] Noisakran S, Onlamoon N, Hsiao HM, Clark KB, Villinger F, Ansari AA, Perng GC. Infection of bone marrow cells by dengue virus in vivo. Experimental Hematology. 2012;**40**(3):250-259

[131] Simon AY, Sutherland MR, Pryzdial EL. Dengue virus binding and replication by platelets. Blood. 2015;**126**(3):378-385

[132] Kar M, Singla M, Chandele A, Kabra SK, Lodha R, Medigeshi GR. Dengue Virus Entry and Replication Does Not Lead to Productive Infection in Platelets. Open Forum Infectious Diseases. 2017;**4**(2):ofx051

[133] Aatonen MT, Öhman T, Nyman TA, Laitinen S, Grönholm M, Siljande PRM. Isolation and characterization of platelet-derived extracellular vesicles. Journal of Extracellular Vesicles. 2014;**3**

[134] Aslam R, Speck ER, Kim M, Crow AR, Bang KW, Nestel FP, Ni H, Lazarus AH, Freedman J, Mint SJW. Platelet toll-like receptor expression modulates lipopolysaccharide-induced thrombocytopenia and tumor necrosis factor-α production in vivo. Blood. 2006;**107**(2):637-641

[135] Shashkin PN, Brown GT, Ghosh A, Marathe GK, McIntyre TM. Lipopolysaccharide is a direct agonist for platelet RNA splicing. The Journal of Immunology. 2008;**181**(5): 3495-3502

[136] Carestia A, Kaufman T, Schattner M. Platelets: New Bricks in the Building of Neutrophil Extracellular Traps. Frontiers in Immunology. 2016;**7**(271)

[137] Peters MJ, Dixon G, Kotowicz KT, Hatch DJ, Heyderman RS, Mint KNJ. Circulating platelet–neutrophil complexes represent a subpopulation of activated neutrophils primed for adhesion, phagocytosis and intracellular killing. British Journal of Haematology. 1999;**106**(2):391-399

[138] Krishnamurti C, Peat RA, Cutting MA, Mint RSW. Platelet adhesion to dengue-2 virus-infected endothelial cells. The American Journal of Tropical Medicine and Hygiene. 2002;**66**(4):435-441

[139] Onlamoon N, Noisakran S, Hsiao HM, Duncan A, Villinger F, Ansari AA, Perng GC. Mint: Dengue virus–induced hemorrhage in a nonhuman primate model. Blood. 2010;**115**(9): 1823-1834

[140] Andrews RK, Arthur JF, Gardiner EE. Mint: Neutrophil extracellular traps (NETs) and the role of platelets in infection. Thrombosis and Haemostasis. 2014;**112**(4):659-665

[141] Butthep P, Bunyaratvej A, Bhamarapravati N. Mint: Dengue virus and endothelial cell: A related phenomenon to thrombocytopenia and granulocytopenia in dengue hemorrhagic fever. The Southeast Asian Journal of Tropical Medicine and Public Health. 1992;**24**:246-249

[142] Chen K, Detwiler TC, Essex DW. Mint: Characterization of protein disulphide isomerase released from activated platelets. British Journal of Haematology. 1995;**90**(2):425-431

[143] Essex DW, Li M. Protein disulphide isomerase mediates platelet aggregation and secretion. British Journal of Haematology. 1999;**104**(3):448-454

[144] Rachman A, Harahap AR, Widhyasih RM. Mint: The role of anti-dengue virus NS-1 and anti-protein disulfide isomerase antibodies on platelet aggregation in secondary dengue infection. Acta Medica Indonesiana. 2013;**45**(1):44-48

[145] Cheng HJ, Lei HY, Lin CF, Luo YH, Wan SW, Liu HS, Yeh TM, Lin YS. Mint: Anti-dengue virus nonstructural protein 1 antibodies recognize protein disulfide isomerase on platelets and inhibit platelet aggregation. Molecular Immunology. 2009;**47**(2):398-406

[146] Nachman RL, Rafii S. Mint: Platelets, petechiae, and preservation of the vascular wall. New England Journal of Medicine. 2008;**359**(12):1261-1270

[147] Michels M, van der Ven AJ, Djamiatun K, Fijnheer R, de Groot PG, Griffioen AW, Sebastian S, Faradz SM, de Mastro Q. Mint: Imbalance of angiopoietin-1 and angiopoetin-2 in severe dengue and relationship with thrombocytopenia, endothelial activation, and vascular stability. The American Journal of Tropical Medicine and Hygiene. 2012;**87**(5):943-946

[148] Trugilho MRO, Hottz ED, Brunoro GVF, Teixeira-Ferreira A, Carvalho PC, Salazar GA, Zimmerman GA, Bozza FA, Bozza PT, Perales J. Mint: Platelet proteome reveals novel pathways of platelet activation and platelet-mediated immunoregulation in dengue. PLoS Pathogens 2017;**13**(5):e1006385

[149] Fragnoud R, Flamand M, Reynier F, Buchy P, Duong V, Pachot A, Paranhos-Baccala G, Bedin F. Mint: Differential proteomic analysis of virus-enriched fractions obtained from plasma pools of patients with dengue fever or severe dengue. BMC Infectious Diseases. 2015;**15**:518

Chapter 3

Not Only Heparin but Also Antibody Induces Thrombocytopenia

Thi-Huong Nguyen

Additional information is available at the end of the chapter

http://dx.doi.org/10.5772/intechopen.73576

Abstract

In the last two decades, heparin was widely used as an anticoagulant. Besides numerous advantages of heparin, some patients with heparin administration suffer from a side effect, the so-called heparin-induced thrombocytopenia (HIT), which can result in thromboses such as deep vein thrombosis, pulmonary embolism, occlusion of a limb artery, acute myocardial infarct, stroke, and a systemic reaction or skin necrosis. The basic on HIT complication have been investigated and led to clinical insights. Recent studies provided detail mechanisms among binding partners in HIT; especially, it has been shown that not only heparin but also a subset of antibody induce thrombocytopenia. In this chapter, insights into both heparin- and antibody-induced thrombocytopenia will be discussed and the novel mechanism of the autoimmune HIT caused by a subset of antibodies will be introduced.

Keywords: heparin-induced thrombocytopenia, HIT, mechanism, binding force, PF4, antibody

1. Introduction

Heparin-induced thrombocytopenia (HIT) as a severe adverse drug effect occurs when patients receive heparin anticoagulant to prevent and treat thromboembolic diseases. Depending on the length of heparin, HIT occurs in ≤5% of patients receiving high molecular weight unfractionated heparin, whereas ≤1% of patients receiving low molecular weight heparin. In HIT, the immune system considers the platelet factor 4 (PF4), which is altered in its conformation after binding to heparin (H), to be "foreign" and the formation of anti-PF4/H antibodies (aPF4/P Abs) occurs. Upon binding to the PF4/H complex, these antibodies activate circulating platelets and other cells. Typically, 5–14 days after heparin exposure, platelet count reduces to <15–20 × 10^9 cells/L (or a > 50% decrease in platelet count). HIT can result in thromboses such as deep vein thrombosis (DVT), pulmonary embolism (PE), occlusion of a limb artery, acute myocardial infarct, stroke, and a systemic reaction or skin necrosis. Importantly, there is also a subset of anti-PF4/Heparin antibodies (aPF4/H Abs) which, in the absence of heparin, can lead to symptomatic thrombocytopenia and excessive vascular thrombosis. The extreme sequela of the aPF4/H Abs is autoimmune HIT, in which individuals develop multiple vessel occlusions without drug exposure.

2. Heparin-induced thrombocytopenia

Heparin-induced thrombocytopenia (HIT) is a distinct clinicopathologic syndrome caused by platelet-activating antibodies that bridge between complexes of platelet factor 4-Heparin (PF4/H) and platelets [1, 2] or endothelial cells [3]. Human platelets are anuclear cell fragments with discoidal shapes of 1–2 μm, originating from the cytoplasm of bone marrow megakaryocytes [4]. Platelets store PF4 (a positively charged tetramer belonging to CXC chemokine family) in their alpha granules. Non-activated platelets release some PF4s (**Figure 1A**) [5]. When patients take anticoagulant polyanions like heparin, some of these heparins bind to PF4s forming ultra large PF4/H complexes (**Figure 1B**). Binding of heparin to PF4 induces a conformational change in PF4s [6–8] which results in an expression of new epitopes. Some patients develop antibodies against these neoepitopes (**Figure 1B**). These human-derived antibodies are defined as anti-PF4/H antibodies (aPF4/P Abs). Each resulting multimolecular complex

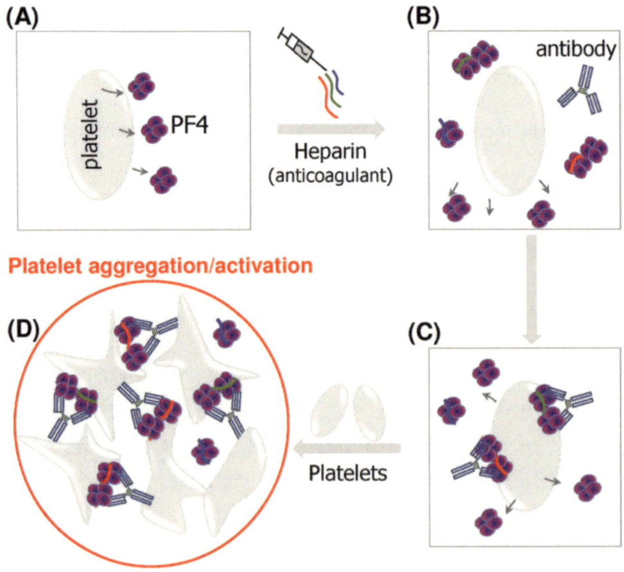

Figure 1. Cartoon illustrates the formation of heparin-induced thrombocytopenia (HIT). (A) Non-activated platelets secrete several PF4s. (B) with heparin exposure, PF4s form ultra large complexes with long heparins that induce conformational changes in PF4s. Some patients develop aPF4/H Abs against PF4 neoepitopes. (C) Human-derived aPF4/H Abs bound PF4/H complexes can adhere to platelet membrane. (D) Fc parts of the antibodies link fcγRIIa receptors on platelet membranes that leads to platelet aggregation/activation. Adapted from [5].

of an aPF4/P Ab to a PF4/H complex contains two platelet binding sites, that is, one is on the PF4/H complexes, and another one is on the Fc part of the IgG which binds to FcγRIIa receptors [9, 10] on platelet membranes (**Figure 1C**). Cross-linking of the platelet Fc receptor results in platelet activation that releases more PF4s and facilitates formation additional ultra large immune complexes. These complexes rapidly recruit other platelets into the prothrombotic process (**Figure 1D**). Activation of platelets leads to the loss of platelets, massive platelet activation and even triggers clotting cascade that results in thrombin generation and increases the risk for vessel occlusions such as venous thrombosis, myocardial infarction or stroke [7, 11, 12]. The binding strength of a blood thrombus has major biological importance. A recent study could determine directly the binding strength between two platelets at single platelet level [13]. The binding force increases proportionally to the degree of platelet activation but reduces with blockade of specific platelet receptors. The method provides major perspectives for testing and improving the biocompatibility of new materials, quantifying the effect of drugs on platelet function, and assessing the mechanical characteristics of acquired/inherited platelet defects.

Heparins are the glycosaminoglycans (GAGs) containing glucosamine residues with a high degree of sulfation that dictates their biological activities [6, 14, 15]. GAGs play an important role in the sequestration of plasmodium falciparum-infected red blood cells in the microvascular endothelium of different tissues [16, 17]. Their pharmacologic activity is mediated by a chemically unique pentasaccharide sequence present in about 30% of all heparin molecules. Heparin behaves like simple entropic spring forces, which is produced by sugar rings of heparin flipping to more energetic and more extended conformations [18, 19]. Both low and high molecular weight heparins are available. The source of high molecular weight unfractionated heparin (UFH) influences the risk of HIT, i.e. bovine UFH is more likely to cause HIT than porcine UFH [20–22]. Besides UFH, the low molecular weight heparins (LMWH) produced from UFH by chemical fractionation, are widely used in clinical practice [23–27]. Due to their shorter chain length, LMWHs show less strong interaction with PF4. UFH and PF4 form ultra large complexes (ULCs) when both are present approximately at an optimal 1:1 ratio. Comparing with UFH, LMWHs form smaller complexes with PF4. ULCs showed a greater capacity to promote platelet activation than small complexes [28]. These differences in complex formation between UFH and LMWHs translate into their risk for inducing HIT in patients. LMWHs induce HIT about 10 times less frequent than UFH, but HIT still randomly occurs during treatment with LMWHs [29–32].

2.1. Boundary between antigenic and non-antigenic heparin

PF4/heparin (or polyanions) complexes can become antigenic or not depend on heparin (or polyanion) characteristics. To expose neoepitopes on PF4s relevant for HIT, at least three bonds between the polyanion and PF4 in the PF4/polyanion complex should be formed [33]. These neoepitopes on the PF4/polyanion complexes then allow binding of the aPF4/H Abs. The binding strength of the single sulfate groups on the polyanion with the PF4 does not differ among polyanions with a different degree of sulfation [33]. The quantity and resulting density of sulfate groups on the polyanion chain determine their molecular effects on PF4 [33]. In particular, the polyanions which bind to PF4 tetramer with less than three sulfate bonds are unable to expose the neoepitope [6, 34]. The results suggest an existence of a boundary between antigenic (risk for HIT) and non-antigenic heparins (non-risk for HIT). This boundary has been determined by applying multiple techniques such as atomic force microscopy-based atomic force microscopy (AFS) [35], isothermal titration calorimetry (ITC) [6], or circular dichroism (CD) spectroscopy in combination with enzyme-linked immunosorbent assay (ELISA) [7] (**Figure 2**).

AFS shows that both numbers of specific rupture events and magnitude of rupture forces rise with an increase of heparin length, suggesting that long heparins form with PF4 more bonds than short ones [35]. A larger variation of the rupture forces for long heparins ≥8-mer compared with short heparins ≤6-mer was observed (**Figure 3A**). The enthalpy obtained by ITC rises with the increase of heparin length and reaches maximal values at ~11-mer (**Figure 3B**) [36]. Combining the results obtained by AFS and ITC, the boundary between non-antigenic and antigenic heparin is determined between 8- to 11-mer. This boundary is further clarified by CD spectroscopy which is sensitive to the secondary structure and folding properties of proteins [37]. For PF4/H interactions, the change in β-sheet content was found to be ≤30% for short heparin and >30% for long heparins (**Figure 3C**). By ELISA, optical density (OD) was ≤0.5 for short heparin, while OD was >0.5 for longer heparins (>8-mer) (**Figure 3C**). The OD of 0.5 is the threshold to determine whether a heparin used in the ELISA was able to support binding of aPF4/H Abs. The combination of β-sheet content and OD values show clearly a dissimilar behavior between short and long heparins (**Figure 3C**).

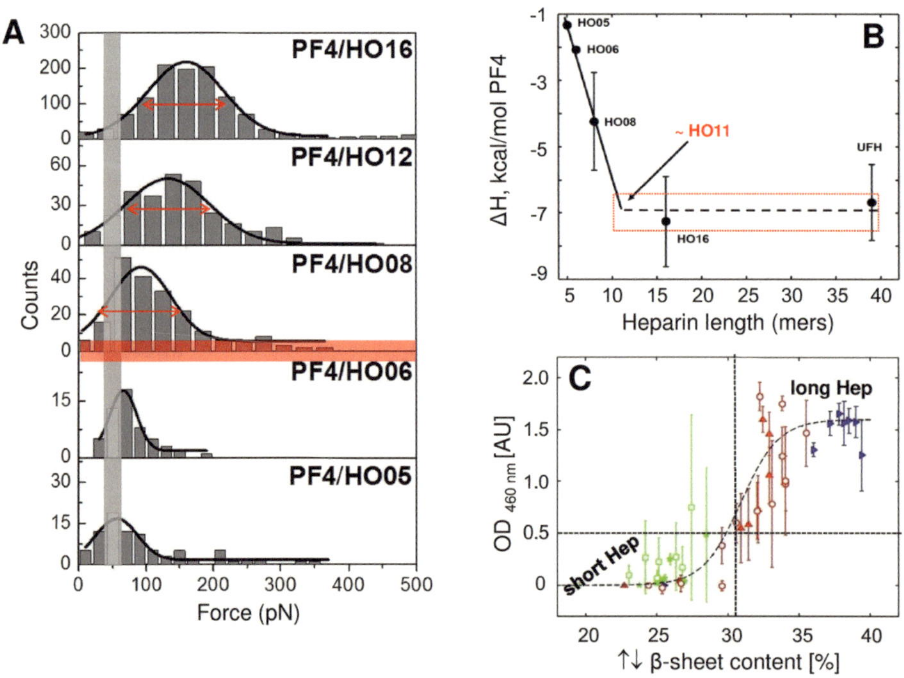

Figure 2. Determination of the boundary between antigenic and non-antigenic heparins. (A) Rupture force histograms fitted by Gaussian distributions show narrow widths (green arrows) for heparins ≤6-mer (HO05, HO06) and wider widths for longer heparins ≥8-mer (HO08, HO012, HO016). (B) ITC demonstrates lower enthalpy for short heparins (black dotted box) and higher enthalpy for long heparins (red-dotted box), while a saturation is found at ~11-mer. (C) Combination of CD spectroscopy and EIA shows that a boundary between short and long heparins is at ~30% ß-sheet contents and OD ~0.5. Overall, the boundary is determined between 8- and 11-mer. Adapted from [8, 35, 48].

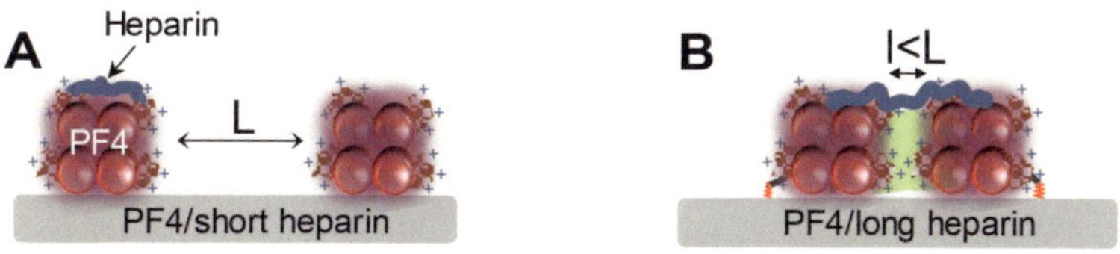

Figure 3. Model describing different binding pathways between short and long heparins when interacting with PF4 tetramers. (A) Depending on heparin length, short heparin can bind to one PF4 tetramer, (B) whereas long heparin bridges two PF4s and forces them closer to each other at a distance $l < L$, merging two hydrophobic surfaces of PF4s (green shaded area). Adapted from [35].

Linking together all the results from AFS, ITC, CD spectroscopy and ELISA, the boundary between antigenic and non-antigenic heparin has been proved between 8- and 11-mer. These findings are particularly important to understand PF4-Heparin binding processes and to develop new heparin-derived drugs with reduced risk for adverse immune reactions. Combination of these techniques allows better characterizing heparin boundary.

2.2. Kinetic properties and binding model of PF4/H complexes

Thermodynamic and kinetic parameters of the ligand-receptor interactions can be obtained by applying the Bell-Evans [38] or the Friddle [39, 40] models. The models show that the faster the molecule is pulled, the higher the rupture force will be measured. For simple ligand-receptor interaction in which multiple interactions are not involved, the rupture force (F) increases proportionally to the logarithmic loading rate. Even though there is some variation in the parameters obtained by these two models, Bell-Evans model is still a powerful tool to determine the kinetics of ligand-receptor interactions [41, 42]. For the PF4/H system, the PF4 tetramer is considered as one antigen or the interaction between heparin and PF4 is formed by a single bond, and therefore, applicable to the Bell-Evans model [35]. Short heparins show higher k_{off} values than long heparins, indicating that PF4/long heparin complexes are more stable than PF4/short heparin complexes (**Table 1**). With binding affinity (K_A) measured by ITC [6], the thermal on-rate ($k_{on} = k_{off} \cdot K_A$) of PF4/H complexes is calculated. The short heparins bind to PF4s with ~10–20 times faster than long heparins [35].

PF4-Heparins interaction is more complex than general ligand-receptor interactions which are attributed to the electrostatic attraction. Based on special features in force-distance curves and the magnitude of PF4/H binding forces, it has been proved that long heparin bound PF4s creating additional PF4-PF4 bonds [35]. Long heparins form two types of bonds with PFs, i.e.

Parameter	HO06	HO12	HO16
k_{off} (s^{-1})	1.64	1.40×10^{-2}	1.10×10^{-4}
k_{on}(M^{-1} s^{-1})	0.41×10^{5}	0.32×10^{4}	0.55×10^{3}
ΔE (k_BT)	−0.49	4.27	9.12

Table 1. Thermodynamic and kinetic parameters of PF4/heparin interactions [35].

(i) PF4-Heparin and (ii) PF4-PF4 bond, whereas short heparins form only one PF4-Heparin bond. Even though the concept of the PF4-PF4 bond, in general, cannot be accepted because PF4s are highly positive proteins, and therefore, strongly repel each other. However, when forming a complex with a highly negative charged heparin, the positive-charged PF4 is probably neutralized that results in a mergence of two hydrophobic PF4 surfaces [34]. Based on these findings, a model for PF4-heparin interaction has been proposed (**Figure 3**). Due to their sizes, the short heparins simply bind to a single PF4 tetramer (**Figure 3A**), whereas the long heparins neutralize positive charges on PF4 tetramers and switch the charges between two PF4 tetramers from a repulsion to an attraction. Heparin reacts as a catalyst that forces two PF4 molecules close to each other within a distance l ($l < L$), resulting in two merged hydrophobic PF4 surfaces (**Figure 3B**). This way of interacting results in the extremely stable PF4/H complexes, especially for long heparins.

A sequence in the formation of PF4/heparin complexes has been identified. When a long heparin comes closely to PF4s, heparin forms first bonds with positively charged clusters on PF4s and then it pulls closely PF4s together to form PF4-PF4 bonds [35].

Based on bond energy (ΔE), quantitative information of bond transitions can be calculated following the study of Wang et al. [43]. The bond transitions of short heparin from the weak positive-charged area on PF4 release energy, whereasPF4-PF4 bonds consume energy [35]. In contrast to short heparin, the bond transitions of long heparins in both cases release energy, while their interactions with the positively charged clusters consume energy (**Table 1**). Based on energy level, PF4-PF4 interaction is attributed to be stronger than the bonds between heparin and non-clusters of positive-charged areas on PF4. However, PF4-PF4 interaction is weaker than the interaction between heparin and clusters of positive charges on PF4.

3. Antibody-induced thrombocytopenia

Immunocomplexes composed of aPF4/P Abs and PF4/polyanion (PF4/P) complexes on the platelet surface induce platelet aggregation via cross-linking FcγRIIA receptors [9, 10]. They also bind to the surface of endothelial cells and monocytes [44–46], inducing procoagulant activity [44, 47]. Heparin-induced thrombocytopenia has been well understood. Recent studies reported that a subset of human-derived autoantibodies in some patients also can induce thrombocytopenia in a heparin-similar manner.

3.1. Human-derived HIT antibodies

All aPF4/P Abs bind to immobilized PF4/P complexes in ELISA [48], but only some of them activate platelets in functional assays, e.g. the heparin-induced platelet activation assay (HIPA) [48] or the serotonin release assay (SRA) [49, 50]. Human-derived aPF4/P Abs compose of three groups, i.e. the antibodies do not activate platelets in HIPA test (group-1 Abs); the antibodies activate platelets in HIPA but require heparin (group-2 Abs); the antibodies activate platelets even without heparin (group-3 Abs) (**Figure 4**). Group-3 Abs developed from patients who had clinical autoimmune HIT, and therefore, they are defined as 'autoantibodies' [51].

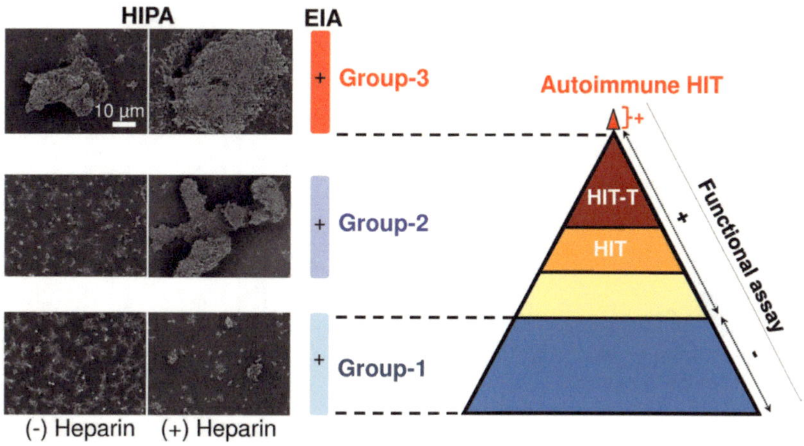

Figure 4. Different reaction patterns of aPF4/H antibodies. (Right) pyramid shows antibodies of three groups, all positive in EIA. Group-1 (blue) do not activate platelets (HIPA -); many Abs belonging to group-2 do not induce HIT (yellow), some induce HIT (gold) and others induce HIT with thrombosis (dark red). Recent studies found an additional small subset of patient's content autoimmune group-3 HIT Abs (red). (Left) visualization of platelet aggregates-induced by different antibody groups imaged by scanning electron microscopy in the presence (+) or absence (−) of heparin: Group-1 abs induce (bottom left) only small aggregates reflecting the background platelet activation; group-2 Abs (middle, left) cause large aggregates only in the presence of heparin; group-3 Abs induce large aggregates even in the absence of heparin. Same scale bar for all images. Adapted from [55].

3.1.1. Characteristics of human-derived HIT antibodies

In contrast to the detailed characterization of the PF4/polyanion complexes, little is known about the features of aPF4/H Abs in the pathogenesis of HIT. Exploring the characteristics of HIT antibodies bears a potential to better understand general mechanisms of antibody-mediated autoimmunity HIT. However, there is a difficulty in subtracting the pathogenic HIT antibody directly from human sera because both pathogenic and non-pathogenic antibodies bind to the PF4/H antigen.

Newman et al. reported that aPF4/P Abs can be purified by PF4-agarose beads [3]. Later in 2000, Amiral et al. described that affinity purification of aPF4/P Abs resulted in a mixture of IgA, IgM, and IgG [52]. In this mixture, only a subset of IgG antibodies activates platelets [49]. Contamination of IgA, IgM, and IgG antibodies will increase the difficulty in characterizing aPF4/P Abs. To overcome this limitation, two-step affinity chromatography has currently established to separate aPF4/H Abs from HIT patients sera. By this method, aPF4/P Abs from sera of patients were successfully isolated for three antibody groups. The purified Abs showed similar characteristics as the original serum in EIA and HIPA. Titrating the antibodies in ELISA, all antibody groups show an increase of OD with increasing antibody concentration (**Figure 5A**). OD values are highest for group-3, followed by group-2 and then group-1 Abs. In the HIPA test, group-1 Abs did not cause platelet aggregation up to a concentration of 89.7 μg/mL; group-2 Abs induced platelet aggregation from concentrations ≥43.5 μg/mL, but only in the presence of heparin; while group-3 Abs induced platelet aggregation from concentrations ≥5.2 μg/mL independently of heparin (**Figure 5B**). This is consistent with previous findings that chondroitin sulfate plays an important role in platelet activation by PF4/P Abs, even in the absence of heparin [53, 54].

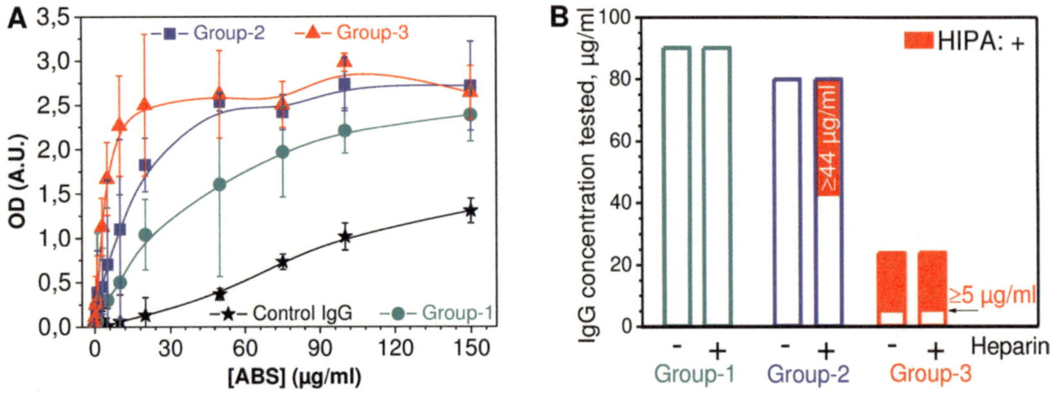

Figure 5. Dose-dependent binding of aPF4/P Abs to PF4/H complexes in EIA and HIPA. (A) EIA shows the lowest OD of control IgG (black) as the background reaction, follow by group-1 (dark cyan), higher for group-2 (blue) and highest for group-3 (red) Abs. (B) HIPA tests show a dependence of platelet aggregation on antibody concentration: Group-1 Abs do not activate platelets, neither in the absence (−), nor in the presence (+) of reviparin up to a concentration of 89.7 μg/mL (dark cyan); group-2 Abs (blue) induced platelet activation (red part) at concentrations ≥44 μg/mL but only in the presence of reviparin; group-3 Abs (red) activated platelets at much lower concentrations (≥5 μg/mL) either in the presence or absence of reviparin. n = 5 sera per group. Adapted from [55].

3.1.2. Binding strength of human-derived HIT antibodies

The binding strength between the antibody and PF4/H complexes is determined by AFS. A single aPF4/H Abs is immobilized on the cantilever and then approach to the PF4/H complexes coated on a solid phase for interacting and measuring of their binding strength. Weakest binding forces were measured for monoclonal antibody KKO mimicking human HIT antibodies (43.6 ± 8.8 pN, gray) and group-1 Abs (44.0 ± 8.1 pN, green), higher for group-2 Abs (60.6 ± 15.4 pN, blue) and highest for group-3 Abs (72.4 ± 26.2 pN, red). Statistics showed no significant difference between KKO and group-1 Abs (p = 0.877), significant difference between group-1 and group-2 Abs (p < 0.001), or between group-2 and group-3 Abs (p = 0.006)) (**Figure 6**) [55].

Group-3 Abs bound to PF4/H complexes with much higher binding energy ($\Delta H = -2.87 \pm 2.06 \times 10^8$ cal/mol) than group-2 Abs ($\Delta H = -2.90 \pm 0.4 \times 10^4$ cal/mol), and their dissociation constant (K_D) (~5.3 nM) was about two orders of magnitude lower than that of group-2 Abs (~1.7×10^2 nM). The binding strength of PF4 to heparin ~150 pN [35] is higher than that between group-3 Abs and PF4/H complexes (mostly lower than 150 pN) [55]. Besides that, the group-3 Abs have a highest binding affinity (k_{off} = 0.12 s^{-1}) as compared with group-1 Abs y (k_{off} = 15.6 s^{-1}), group-2 Abs (k_{off} = 2.0 s^{-1}), or KKO (k_{off} = 2.2 s^{-1}). The lowest thermal off-rate specify that multiplexes induced by PF4/H complexes with group-3 Abs are more stable than those formed with other antibody groups. Furthermore, KKO and group-1 Abs contain antibodies with similar characteristics, and therefore, they interacted rather uniformly with PF4/H complexes. This has been clarified by obtaining the relatively small differences among the rupture forces (<60 pN, **Figure 6A-B**) measured from different cantilevers. However, group-2 Abs contain different types of antibodies as observed by a large variation of all binding forces (~40% exceeded 60 pN). For group-3 Abs, the variation of binding force is even higher than that of group-2 Abs as shown by ~44% of all binding forces ≥60 pN and ~15%

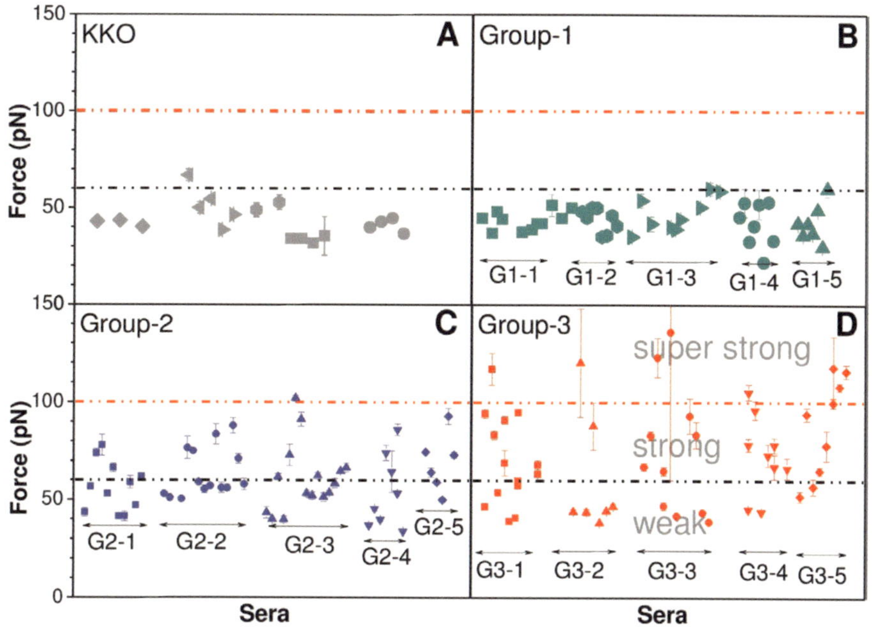

Figure 6. Binding characteristics of aPF4/H Abs. Each dot shows the mean and standard error of the rupture force for each respective antibody from five sera per group. (A) KKO and (B) group-1 Abs bind to PF4/H complexes with a binding strength mostly ≤60 pN (black dotted line), while (C) group-2 and (C) group-3 Abs consist of Abs with different binding forces. (D) a subset of group-3 Abs binds to PF4/H complexes with rupture forces higher than 100 pN (red-dotted line). Adapted from [55].

even exceeded 100 pN. The low variability in binding forces of KKO and group-1 Abs has been attributed to the fact that they contain homogeneous antibodies, whereas the patient's sera such as group-2 and group-3 Abs contained polyclonal mixtures of aPF4/P Abs differently reactive. Among these human-derived Abs, it has been proved that the group-2 contains also antibodies reacting like group-1 Abs, while group-3 is highly complicated as it composes of not only antibodies reacting like group-1 and group-2 Abs but also some additional super strong reactive antibodies. The aPF4/H Abs show different reactivity patterns under various pH and ionic strength conditions [56].

3.1.3. Autoimmune antibodies cluster PF4

The autoimmune group-3 Abs activate platelets in the absence of polyanions because they can self-cluster PF4 to form PF4/group-3 antibody complexes without the need of heparin [55]. This characteristic of autoimmune group-3 Abs has been proved by various methodologies:

First, the autoimmune group-3 Abs could be purified from the patient's sera using a PF4-column (instead of the PF4/H column). Hardly any PF4/P Abs were obtained from control and group-1 sera; group-2 sera showed a minimally increased IgG yield. When these antibodies are concentrated to 50 μg/ml, only antibodies purified from group-3 sera activated platelets in the HIPA. The results indicate that group-3 sera contain antibodies with PF4 specificity, which activate platelets.

Next, only autoantibodies (group-3) show strong interaction with PF4 alone by ITC. When the antibodies were tested at the same concentration of 62.5 nM, KKO and group-2 Abs did not interact with PF4, while group-3 Abs interacted strongly. As the interaction between group-3 Abs and PF4 alone showed two binding sites (stoichiometry $n = C_{ABS}/C_{PF4} = 0.53 \pm 0.003$), these Abs can cluster two PF4 molecules. Increasing antibody concentration did not improve binding of KKO to PF4 whereas group-2 Abs weakly interacted with PF4. However, the binding energy released by group-2 Abs is only 0.1% compared to that of group-3 Abs.

Consistently, PF4 or PF4/H EIA show that group-3 Abs bound quite strong to PF4 while other antibodies did not even though all Abs bound much stronger to PF4/H complexes than to PF4 alone. By AFS, group-1 and group-2 Abs showed much less binding events to PF4 than to PF4/H complexes, while the super-reactive group-3 Abs showed similar bindings. In addition, the interaction forces of group-3 Abs purified via a PF4-column with PF4/H complexes showed the highest range of binding forces (~100 pN). These results again indicate that group-3 Abs bind strongly to PF4 alone independently from heparin, while bindings of group-1 and group-2 Abs are heparin-dependent.

By dynamic light scattering (DLS), group-3 Abs formed the largest complexes with PF4 as compared to other antibody groups with even larger size than PF4/H complexes further indicate that group-3 Abs can cluster PF4.

The binding energy generated by the interaction of group-3 Abs with PF4 in the ITC experiments ($\Delta H = -3.5 \pm 0.86 \times 10^7$cal/mol) is much higher than the energy released when a 16-mer heparin interacts with PF4 ($\Delta H = -7.26 \pm 1.36 \times 10^3$ cal/mol) [6]. As 16-mer heparin can force two PF4 molecules together, based on their high energy release, group-3 Abs most probably also can force two PF4 tetramers together. In addition, the negative entropy of the reaction ($\Delta S = -11.7 \pm 2.8 \times 10^4$ cal/mol. K) is attributed to PF4 conformational change when forming complexes with the group-3 Abs. By DLS, the size complexes formed by PF4 and group-3 Abs increases significantly when the group-2 Abs are added, indicating that group-3 Abs, induce a conformational change in PF4 and the resulting PF4/group-3 antibody complexes allow binding of group-2 Abs in the same way as polyanions do.

Altogether, PF4 form large complexes with heparin and allow group-2 Abs bind and induce platelet aggregation/activation (**Figure 7A-C**). Importantly, a subset of group-3 Abs cluster PF4 and the resulting PF4/Group-3 antibody complexes also allow binding of group-2 Abs and enhance platelet aggregation/activation even stronger than heparins do as shown by tighter and denser aggregates (**Figure 7D-F**).

3.2. HIT-like antibodies

Many studies in HIT have been performed with human aPF4/P Abs isolated from patient plasma because only one monoclonal antibody (KKO) mimicking human HIT antibodies did exist until recently [57]. KKO activates platelets [58] and monocytes [59] *in vitro* and *in vivo* by cross-linking FcγRIIa. KKO has been used to unravel the pathogenesis of HIT and is the basis for a recently FDA approved plasma-based antigen assay (HIT-HemosIL) for detection of PF4/P antibodies [60, 61]. KKO mimics the biological activity of human aPF4/P Abs [62]

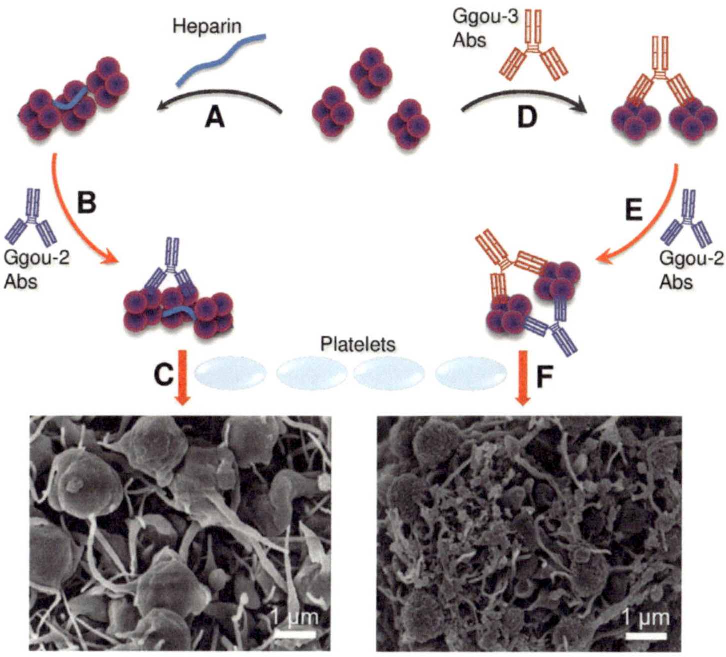

Figure 7. Group-3 Abs cluster PF4 and enhance platelet activation. (A) PF4 form large complexes with heparin and the resulting PF4/H complexes allow (B) group-2 Abs bind and (C) induce platelet aggregation/activation. (D) a subset of group-3 Abs cluster PF4 forming PF4/Group-3 antibody complexes which also (E) allow binding of group-2 Abs and (F) enhance platelet aggregation/activation evidenced by tighter and denser aggregates compared to (C). Adapted from [55].

and has been used to understand the binding characteristics of an antibody recognizing PF4/P complexes and activating platelets [62, 63]. Binding of a non-HIT antibody RTO to PF4 monomers prevents PF4 tetramerization and inhibits KKO and human HIT IgG-induced platelet activation/aggregation in vitro, and thrombus progression in vivo. The probability and the interaction force of KKO binding to PF4 are much greater than those of RTO, while KKO/PF4 dissociation rate was approximately 10-fold slower than RTO/PF4 [62, 63], indicating that KKO binds stronger than RTO and KKO/PF4 complexes are more stable than RTO/PF4.

KKO interacts with PF4/H complexes coated platelets with ~4-fold higher forces than with PF4/H complexes coated on a solid phase, while RTO shows only a minor change [64]. The different binding forces strongly indicate that PF4 and PF4/H complexes either expose different epitopes or allow better access of platelet-activating Abs to their epitope when PF4 bound to the platelet surface compared to the presentation of PF4/H complexes on a solid phase. Most probably, PF4/H complexes exhibited the antigenic site differently depending on the bound substrates [53]. The findings provide an explanation for the surprising observation that KKO interact relatively weak when PF4/H complexes are immobilized on a solid phase [55], while it strongly activates platelets in functional assays. It is unresolved, which additional binding partners on the platelet surface interfere with the conformational change or different presentations of PF4/H complexes. Nevertheless, chondroitin sulfate [53] and polyphosphates [65] are potential candidates, as they interact with PF4.

However, KKO is a mouse IgG2b antibody (an absent subclass in humans) [66], while the platelet-activating aPF4/P Abs present in HIT plasma samples are predominantly IgG1. KKO behaves differently from human aPF4/P Abs, i.e. it binds only weakly to PF4/H complexes coated on a solid phase [64]. Recently, a chimeric monoclonal aPF4/H Abs with a human Fc fragment (5B9) has been developed [67]. The 5B9 antibody has been demonstrated to fully mimic the cellular effects of human HIT Abs [10, 68].

4. Diagnosis of HIT

Immunologic assays, such as polytypic ELISA, IgG-specific ELISA, and particle gel immunoassay (PGI) have a sensitivity, are widely used to detect aPF4/H Abs in the diluted human sera because of their high sensitivity (≥95%) and the fast turn-around. However, only ~50% of aPF4/H Abs detected by antigen tests are clinically irrelevant. The results from positive immunologic assays may lead to an overtreatment for HIT that can result in serious consequences, such as venous limb gangrene or fatal hemorrhage [69]. However, immunologic assays are still powerful tools to rule-out patients with HIT. The cut-off optical intensity (OD) in ELISA was defined at 0.5. An ELISA test showing OD > 0.5 is normally suspected to contain aPF4/H Abs. To increase the specificity of clinically relevant antibodies, a higher OD cut-off for the antigen tests (e.g. OD > 1.0) had been suggested [70].

Even though functional assays such as by serotonin release assay (SRA) [71] or HIPA [72] have a sensitivity of ~90% which is slightly lower than the immunologic assays, these tests show a much better specificity of over 90%. For the better identifying HIT, it is recommended that a positive PF4/H ELISA should prompt confirmatory testing by functional assays [73]. However, the functional assays are only available in specialized laboratories and not available in many countries. Therefore, many physicians rely on the results of antigen tests, especially for the first days after clinical suspicion of HIT has been raised until the results of the functional assay is reported.

Besides immunologic assays and functional assays, the chemiluminescent immunoassays such as HemosIL AcuStar HIT-IgG and HemosIL AcuStar HIT-Ab have been recently introduced. These methods are relatively faster (~30 minutes) than the immunologic assays (hours) and showed extremely high sensitivity (~100%) [74]. The assays seem to be ideal for ruling out HIT. Another study used a colorimetric test to detect HIT based on the interaction between platelets and tetrazolium-based indicator dye [75]. The authors reported the quality of detecting HIT is from 96 to 100% agreement with the functional assay C-SRA.

5. Conclusion

Not only heparin but also autoimmune antibodies induce thrombocytopenia. Large antigenic complexes formed between PF4 and either heparin or antibody activate platelets, cause a prothrombotic and result in a variety of thromboembolic and systemic consequences. In autoimmune HIT, aPF4/P Abs activate platelets in the absence of heparin. These antibodies are highly reactive. They can self-cluster PF4-molecules forming antigenic complexes and allow binding of otherwise aPF4/P Abs. The resulting immunocomplexes induce massive platelet activation in the absence of heparin. The source and length of heparins play an important role in inducing thrombocytopenia. Improvement of heparin quality together with discovering new non-heparin drugs should be highly desirable. Patients who are suspected of HIT need to be immediately stopped heparin exposure and switched to an alternative anticoagulant. Regarding patients with antibody-induced thrombocytopenia, the level of complication is much higher than the general heparin-induced thrombocytopenia. To date, these human-derived antibodies are hardly controlled, and therefore, efforts in the field would be appreciated. Clinical tests for detecting HIT antibodies as well as autoimmune HIT antibodies must be improved to achieve an appropriate identification of clinical HIT patients.

Acknowledgements

This work was supported by the Deutsche Forschungsgemeinschaft (DFG, Germany) (NG 133/1-1).

Conflict of interest

The authors declare no competing financial interests.

Author details

Thi-Huong Nguyen

Address all correspondence to: nguyent@uni-greifswald.de

Institute of Immunology and Transfusion Medicine, University Medicine Greifswald, Greifswald, Germany

References

[1] Greinacher A. Heparin-induced thrombocytopenia. The New England Journal of Medicine. 2015;**373**(19):1883-1884

[2] Warkentin TE, Greinacher A. Heparin-Induced Thrombocytopenia. 4th ed. CRC Press; 2013

[3] Blank M, Shoenfeld Y, Tavor S, Praprotnik S, Boffa MC, Weksler B, Walenga MJ, Amiral J, Eldor A. Anti-platelet factor 4/heparin antibodies from patients with heparin-induced thrombocytopenia provoke direct activation of microvascular endothelial cells. International Immunology. 2002;**14**(2):121-129

[4] Michelson AD. Platelets. 3rd ed. Academic Press/Elsevier; 2013

[5] Nguyen TH. Single-molecule force spectroscopy applied to heparin-induced thrombocytopenia. Journal of Molecular Recognition. 2016

[6] Petitou M, van Boeckel CA. A synthetic antithrombin iii binding pentasaccharide is now a drug! What comes next?, Angewandte Chemie. 2004;**43**(24):3118-3133

[7] Jackson SP. The growing complexity of platelet aggregation. Blood. 2007;**109**(12):5087-5095

[8] Brandt S, Krauel K, Gottschalk KE, Renne T, Helm CA, Greinacher A, Block S. Characterisation of the conformational changes in platelet factor 4 induced by polyanions: Towards in vitro prediction of antigenicity. Thrombosis and Haemostasis. 2014;**112**(1):53-64

[9] Kelton JG, Sheridan D, Santos A, Smith J, Steeves K, Smith C, Brown C, Murphy WG. Heparin-induced thrombocytopenia - laboratory studies. Blood. 1988;**72**(3):925-930

[10] Rollin J, Pouplard C, Gruel Y. Risk factors for heparin-induced thrombocytopenia: Focus on fc gamma receptors. Thrombosis and Haemostasis. 2016;**116**(5):799-805

[11] Whiteheart SW. Platelet granules: Surprise packages. Blood. 2011;**118**(5):1190-1191

[12] Sixma JJ, Wester J. The hemostatic plug. Seminars in Hematology. 1977;**14**(3):265-299

[13] Nguyen TH, Palankar R, Bui VC, Medvedev N, Greinacher A, Delcea M. Rupture forces among human blood platelets at different degrees of activation. Scientific Reports-UK. 2016;**6**:1-12. Article ID: 25402

[14] Warkentin TE, Kelton JG. Heparin-induced thrombocytopenia. Annual Review of Medicine. 1989;**40**:31-44

[15] Powell AK, Yates EA, Fernig DG, Turnbull JE. Interactions of heparin/heparan sulfate with proteins: Appraisal of structural factors and experimental approaches. Glycobiology. 2004;**14**(4):17R-30R

[16] Valle-Delgado JJ, Urban P, Fernandez-Busquets X. Demonstration of specific binding of heparin to plasmodium falciparum-infected vs. non-infected red blood cells by single-molecule force spectroscopy. Nanoscale. 2013;**5**(9):3673-3680

[17] Laremore TN, Zhang F, Dordick JS, Liu J, Linhardt RJ. Recent progress and applications in glycosaminoglycan and heparin research. Current Opinion in Chemical Biology. 2009;**13**(5-6):633-640

[18] Marszalek PE, Oberhauser AF, Li H, Fernandez JM. The force-driven conformations of heparin studied with single molecule force microscopy. Biophysical Journal. 2003; **85**(4):2696-2704

[19] Lee G, Nowak W, Jaroniec J, Zhang QM, Marszalek PE. Molecular dynamics simulations of forced conformational transitions in 1,6-linked polysaccharides. Biophysical Journal. 2004;**87**(3):1456-1465

[20] Bailey RT Jr, Ursick JA, Heim KL, Hilleman DE, Reich JW. Heparin-associated thrombocytopenia: A prospective comparison of bovine lung heparin, manufactured by a new process, and porcine intestinal heparin. Drug Intelligence & Clinical Pharmacy. 1986; **20**(5):374-378

[21] Francis JL, Palmer GJ, 3rd RM, Drexler A. Comparison of bovine and porcine heparin in heparin antibody formation after cardiac surgery. The Annals of Thoracic Surgery. 2003;**75**(1):17-22

[22] Green D, Martin GJ, Shoichet SH, Debacker N, Bomalaski JS, Lind RN. Thrombocytopenia in a prospective, randomized, double-blind trial of bovine and porcine heparin. The American Journal of the Medical Sciences. 1984;**288**(2):60-64

[23] Lee JC, Lu XA, Kulkarni SS, Wen YS, Hung SC. Synthesis of heparin oligosaccharides. Journal of the American Chemical Society. 2004;**126**(2):476-477

[24] Codee JDC, Stubba B, Schiattarella M, Overkleeft HS, van Boeckel CAA, van Boom JH, van der Marel GA. A modular strategy toward the synthesis of heparin-like oligosaccharides using monomeric building blocks in a sequential glycosylation strategy. Journal of the American Chemical Society. 2005;**127**(11):3767-3773

[25] de Paz JL, Noti C, Seeberger PH. Microarrays of synthetic heparin oligosaccharides, Journal of the American Chemical Society. 2006;**128**(9):2766-2767

[26] Polat T, Wong CH. Anomeric reactivity-based one-pot synthesis of heparin-like oligosaccharides. Journal of the American Chemical Society. 2007;**129**(42):12795-12800

[27] Xu YM, Cai C, Chandarajoti K, Hsieh PH, Li LY, Pham TQ, Sparkenbaugh EM, Sheng JZ, Key NS, Pawlinski R, Harris EN, Linhardt RJ, Liu J. Homogeneous low-molecular-weight heparins with reversible anticoagulant activity. Nature Chemical Biology. 2014; **10**(4):248-250

[28] Rauova L, Poncz M, McKenzie SE, Reilly MP, Arepally G, Weisel JW, Nagaswami C, Cines DB, Sachais BS. Ultralarge complexes of pf4 and heparin are central to the pathogenesis of heparin-induced thrombocytopenia. Blood. 2005;**105**(1):131-138

[29] Warkentin TE, Levine MN, Roberts RS, Gent M, Horsewood P, Kelton JG. Heparin-induced thrombocytopenia is more common with unfractionated heparin than with low-molecular-weight heparin. Thrombosis and Haemostasis. 1993;**69**(6):911-911

[30] Linhardt RJ, Liu J. Synthetic heparin. Current Opinion in Pharmacology. 2012;**12**(2):217-219

[31] Warkentin TE, Maurer BT, Aster RH. Heparin-induced thrombocytopenia associated with fondaparinux. New England Journal of Medicine. 2007;**356**(25):2653-2654

[32] Martel N, Lee J, Wells PS. Risk for heparin-induced thrombocytopenia. With unfractionated and low-molecular-weight heparin thromboprophylaxis: A meta-analysis. Blood. 2005;**106**(8):2710-2715

[33] Block S, Greinacher A, Helm CA, Delcea M. Characterization of bonds formed between platelet factor 4 and negatively charged drugs using single molecule force spectroscopy. Soft Matter. 2014;**10**(16):2775-2784

[34] Humbert M, Sitbon O, Chaouat A, Bertocchi M, Habib G, Gressin V, Yaici A, Weitzenblum E, Cordier JF, Chabot F, Dromer C, Pison C, Reynaud-Gaubert M, Haloun A, Laurent M, Hachulla E, Cottin V, Degano B, Jais X, Montani D, Souza R, Simonneau G. Survival in patients with idiopathic, familial, and anorexigen-associated pulmonary arterial hypertension in the modern management era. Circulation. 2010;**122**(2):156-163

[35] Nguyen TH, Greinacher A, Delcea M. Quantitative description of thermodynamic and kinetic properties of the platelet factor 4/heparin bonds. Nanoscale. 2015;**7**(22):10130-10139

[36] Saboury AA. A review on the ligand binding studies by isothermal titration calorimetry. Journal of the Iranian Chemical Society. 2006;**3**(1):1-21

[37] Greenfield NJ. Using circular dichroism spectra to estimate protein secondary structure. Nature Protocols. 2006;**1**(6):2876-2890

[38] Evans E, Ritchie K. Dynamic strength of molecular adhesion bonds. Biophysical Journal. 1997;**72**(4):1541-1555

[39] Friddle RW, Noy A, De Yoreo JJ. Interpreting the widespread nonlinear force spectra of intermolecular bonds. Proceedings of National Academy of Sciences USA. 2012; **109**(34):13573-13578

[40] Noy A, Friddle RW. Practical single molecule force spectroscopy: How to determine fundamental thermodynamic parameters of intermolecular bonds with an atomic force microscope. Methods. 2013;**60**(2):142-150

[41] P. Tripathi, A. Beaussart, D. Alsteens, V. Dupres, I. Claes, I. von Ossowski, W. M. de Vos, A. Palva, S. Lebeer, J. Vanderleyden and Y. F. Dufrene, Adhesion and nanomechanics of pili from the probiotic lactobacillus rhamnosus gg, ACS Nano **7** (2013), no. 4, 3685-3697

[42] Hinterdorfer P, Dufrene YF. Detection and localization of single molecular recognition events using atomic force microscopy. Nature Methods. 2006;**3**(5):347-355

[43] Wang B, Xu B. Transition model for ricin-aptamer interactions with multiple pathways and energy barriers. Physical Review. E, Statistical, Nonlinear, and Soft Matter Physics. 2014;**89**(2):022720

[44] Cines DB, Tomaski A, Tannenbaum S. Immune endothelial-cell injury in heparin-associated thrombocytopenia. New England Journal of Medicine. 1987;**316**(10):581-589

[45] Arepally GM, Mayer IM. Antibodies from patients with heparin-induced thrombocytopenia stimulate monocytic cells to express tissue factor and secrete interleukin-8. Blood. 2001;**98**(4):1252-1254

[46] Tutwiler V, Madeeva D, Ahn HS, Andrianova I, Hayes V, Zheng XL, Cines DB, McKenzie SE, Poncz M, Rauova L. Platelet transactivation by monocytes promotes thrombosis in heparin-induced thrombocytopenia. Blood. 2016;**127**(4):464-472

[47] Greinacher A, Eichler P, Lubenow N, Kwasny H, Luz M. Heparin-induced thrombocytopenia with thromboembolic complications: Meta-analysis of 2 prospective trials to assess the value of parenteral treatment with lepirudin and its therapeutic aptt range. Blood. 2000;**96**(3):846-851

[48] Kreimann M, Brandt S, Krauel K, Block S, Helm CA, Weitschies W, Greinacher A, Delcea M. Binding of anti-platelet factor 4/heparin antibodies depends on the thermodynamics of conformational changes in platelet factor 4. Blood. 2014;**124**(15):2442-2449

[49] Warkentin TE. Heparin-induced thrombocytopenia. Current Opinion in Critical Care. 2015;**21**(6):576-585

[50] Warkentin TE, Greinacher A, Gruel Y, Aster RH, Chong BH, scientific, t. standardization committee of the international society on and haemostasis. Laboratory testing for heparin-induced thrombocytopenia: A conceptual framework and implications for diagnosis. Journal of Thrombosis and Haemostasis. 2011;**9**(12):2498-2500

[51] Warkentin TE, Basciano PA, Knopman J, Bernstein RA. Spontaneous heparin-induced thrombocytopenia syndrome: 2 new cases and a proposal for defining this disorder. Blood. 2014;**123**(23):3651-3654

[52] Amiral J, Pouplard C, Vissac AM, Walenga JM, Jeske W, Gruel Y. Affinity purification of heparin-dependent antibodies to platelet factor 4 developed in heparin-induced thrombocytopenia: Biological characteristics and effects on platelet activation. British Journal of Haematology. 2000;**109**(2):336-341

[53] Padmanabhan A, Jones CG, Bougie DW, Curtis BR, McFarland JG, Wang DM, Aster RH. Heparin-independent, pf4-dependent binding of hit antibodies to platelets: Implications for hit pathogenesis. Blood. 2015;**125**(1):155-161

[54] Cines DB, Rauova L, Arepally G, Reilly MP, McKenzie SE, Sachais BS, M P. Heparin-induced thrombocytopenia: An autoimmune disorder regulated through dynamic autoantigen assembly/disassembly. Journal of Clinical Apheresis. 2007;**22**(1):31-36

[55] Nguyen TH, Medvedev N, Delcea M, Greinacher A. Anti-platelet factor 4/polyanion antibodies mediate a new mechanism of autoimmunity. Nature Communications. 2017; **8**:14945

[56] Nguyen TH, Greinacher A. Effect of ph and ionic strength on the binding strength of anti-pf4/polyanion antibodies. European Biophysics Journal (EBJ). 2017;**46**:795-801

[57] Reilly MP, Taylor SM, Hartman NK, Arepally GM, Sachais BS, Cines DB, Poncz M, McKenzie SE. Heparin-induced thrombocytopenia/thrombosis in a transgenic mouse model requires human platelet factor 4 and platelet activation through fc gamma riia. Blood. 2001;**98**(8):2442-2447

[58] Rauova L, Zhai L, Kowalska MA, Arepally GM, Cines DB, Poncz M. Role of platelet surface pf4 antigenic complexes in heparin-induced thrombocytopenia pathogenesis: Diagnostic and therapeutic implications. Blood. 2006;**107**(6):2346-2353

[59] Kasthuri RS, Glover SL, Jonas W, McEachron T, Pawlinski R, Arepally GM, Key NS, Mackman N. Pf4/heparin-antibody complex induces monocyte tissue factor expression and release of tissue factor positive microparticles by activation of fc gamma ri. Blood. 2012;**119**(22):5285-5293

[60] Jourdy Y, Nougier C, Rugeri L, Bordet JC, Sobas F, Negrier C. Prospective evaluation of automatized pf4/heparin immunoassays hemosil hit-ab (pf4-h) for the diagnosis of heparin-induced thrombocytopenia. International Journal of Laboratory Hematology. 2015;**37**(2):244-252

[61] Althaus K, Hron G, Strobel U, Abbate R, Rogolino A, Davidson S, Greinacher A, Bakchoul T. Evaluation of automated immunoassays in the diagnosis of heparin induced thrombocytopenia. Thrombosis Research. 2013;**131**(3):E85-E90

[62] Sachais BS, Litvinov RI, Yarovoi SV, Rauova L, Hinds JL, Rux AH, Arepally GM, Poncz M, Cuker A, Weisel JW, Cines DB. Dynamic antibody-binding properties in the pathogenesis of hit. Blood. 2012;**120**(5):1137-1142

[63] Litvinov RI, Yarovoi SV, Rauova L, Barsegov V, Sachais BS, Rux AH, Hinds JL, Arepally GM, Cines DB, Weisel JW. Distinct specificity and single-molecule kinetics characterize the interaction of pathogenic and non-pathogenic antibodies against platelet factor 4-heparin complexes with platelet factor 4. The Journal of Biological Chemistry. 2013; **288**(46):33060-33070

[64] Nguyen TH, Greinacher A. Platelet factor 4/heparin complexes present their epitopes differently on a solid phase system than on the platelet surface. Blood. 2017

[65] Yarovoi SV, Cines DB, Zaitsev SV, Lebedeva T, Rauova L, Poncz M, Arepally GM, Khandelwal S, et al. Polyphosphate/platelet factor 4 complexes can mediate heparin-independent platelet activation in heparin-induced thrombocytopenia. Blood Advances. 2016;**1**:62-72

[66] Thauvin-Robinet C, Munck A, Huet F, de Becdelievre A, Jimenez C, Lalau G, Gautier E, Rollet J, Flori J, Nove-Josserand R, Soufir JC, Haloun A, Hubert D, Houssin E, Bellis G, Rault G, David A, Janny L, Chiron R, Rives N, Hairion D, Collignon P, Valeri A, Karsenty G, Rossi A, Audrezet MP, Ferec C, Leclerc J, Georges M, Claustres M, Bienvenu T, Gerard B, Boisseau P, Cabet-Bey F, Cheillan D, Feldmann D, Clavel C, Bieth E, Iron A, Simon-Bouy B, Izard V, Steffann J, Viville S, Costa C, Drouineaud V, Fauque P, Binquet C, Bonithon-Kopp C, Morris MA, Faivre L, Goossens M, Roussey M, Girodon E. p. A. H. collaborating working group on, Cftr p. Arg 117 his associated with cbavd and other cftr-related disorders. Journal of Medical Genetics. 2013;**50**(4):220-227

[67] Morio F, Aubin GG, Danner-Boucher I, Haloun A, Sacchetto E, Garcia-Hermoso D, Bretagne S, Miegeville M, Le Pape P. High prevalence of triazole resistance in aspergillus fumigatus, especially mediated by tr/l98h, in a french cohort of patients with cystic fibrosis. The Journal of Antimicrobial Chemotherapy. 2012;**67**(8):1870-1873

[68] Grossi O, Horeau-Langlard D, Agard C, Haloun A, Lefebvre M, Neel A, Hamidou MA. Low-dose methotrexate in pah related to t-cell large granular lymphocyte leukaemia. The European Respiratory Journal. 2012;**39**(2):493-494

[69] Smythe MA, Warkentin TE, Woodhouse AL, Zakalik D. Venous limb gangrene and fatal hemorrhage: Adverse consequences of hit "overdiagnosis" in a patient with antiphospholipid syndrome. American Journal of Hematology. 2011;**86**(2):188-191

[70] Nagler M, Bachmann LM. H. ten Cate and A. ten Cate-Hoek, Diagnostic value of immunoassays for heparin-induced thrombocytopenia: A systematic review and meta-analysis, Blood. 2016;**127**(5):546-557

[71] Warkentin TE. Laboratory testing for heparin-induced thrombocytopenia. Journal of Thrombosis and Thrombolysis. 2000;**10**:S35-S45

[72] Greinacher A. Heparin-induced thrombocytopenia. New England Journal of Medicine. 2015;**373**(3):252-261

[73] Warkentin TE. n. Vol.1, (September 2002), pp.63-72. Heparin-induced thrombocytopenia. Current Hematology Reports. 2002

[74] Legnani C, Cini M, Pili C, Boggian O, Frascaro M, Palareti G. Evaluation of a new automated panel of assays for the detection of anti-pf4/heparin antibodies in patients suspected of having heparin-induced thrombocytopenia. Thrombosis and Haemostasis. 2010;**104**(2):402-409

[75] Prechel MM, Escalante V, Drenth AF, Walenga JM. A colorimetric, metabolic dye reduction assay detects highly activated platelets: Application in the diagnosis of heparin-induced thrombocytopenia. Platelets. 2012;**23**(1):69-80

Chapter 4

Antiphospholipid Syndrome and Thrombocytopenia

Klara Gadó and Gyula Domján

Additional information is available at the end of the chapter

http://dx.doi.org/10.5772/intechopen.72509

Abstract

Antiphospholipid syndrome is characterised by arterial and venous thromboembolic events and pregnancy morbidity (mainly, recurrent foetal losses), in the presence of antiphospholipid antibodies. Diagnosis is based on the presence of at least one laboratory and at least one clinical manifestation of antiphospholipid syndrome. There are also so-called "non-criteria" clinical features, and thrombocytopenia is one of the most important among them. Thrombocytopenia has been reported with a prevalence between 30 and 46% among patients with antiphospholipid syndrome. The pathogenesis of thrombocytopenia related to antiphospholipid antibodies is not absolutely clear. Binding of antiphospholipid antibodies to platelets and the promotion of platelet activation and aggregation thus thrombus formation must be an important mechanism as well as the immune-mediated clearance of platelets. Thrombocytopenia in antiphospholipid syndrome is usually mild and does not require clinical intervention. The presence of thrombocytopenia in patients with antiphospholipid syndrome is typically associated not with haemorrhagic complications, rather it can trigger thrombotic events. Other causes of thrombocytopenia, such as TTP, SLE, MDS, and ITP should be excluded. As thrombocytopenia is usually mild and it predicts later thrombosis, patients may be given platelet aggregation inhibitors and/or anticoagulant therapy. Anti-thrombotic treatment should be stopped only in case of severe thrombocytopenia.

Keywords: antiphospholipid syndrome, APS, antiphospholipid antibody, thrombocytopenia, thrombosis, SLE, pregnancy

1. About antiphospholipid syndrome

Antiphospholipid syndrome (APS) is characterised by arterial and venous thromboembolic events and pregnancy morbidity (mainly, recurrent foetal losses), in the presence of antiphospholipid antibodies (aPLs). APS (or Hughes' syndrome) was first described by GR Hughes in 1983 [1]. APS is a non-inflammatory autoimmune disease, or autoimmune thrombotic disorder, because autoantibodies are generated against different epitopes of the participant of the coagulation system (mainly against phospholipid-binding proteins) that result in thrombosis. These antiphospholipid antibodies are a heterogeneous group of autoantibodies. Lupus anticoagulant (LA), anti-cardiolipin antibodies (ACA) and anti-β2 glycoprotein 1 (aβ2GPI) are the most important among them [2].

APS may be a secondary disease, as it frequently associates to systemic autoimmune diseases such as SLE and also to malignant lymphoproliferative diseases and chronic hepatic disorders [3]. On the contrary, APS can appear without any underlying disease, and in this case, it is called primary antiphospholipid syndrome.

Neurologic involvement in APS is common and can be manifested by headaches, memory impairment, dizziness, epilepsy and blurred vision, but the most common presentations are transient ischaemic attacks and ischaemic strokes. Some of them are not thrombotic manifestations but are generated by connection of aPL antibodies and an antigen in the nervous system [4].

There is a special form of APS: the obstetric antiphospholipid syndrome (OAPS). It is characterised clinically only by obstetrical morbidity: at least two unexplained miscarriages, three non-consecutive miscarriages, preeclampsia, placental abruption, foetal growth restriction, stillbirth, premature birth, or two or more unexplained in vitro fertilisation failures [5, 6].

Catastrophic antiphospholipid syndrome (CAPS) is rare, but very serious form of APS. The mortality rate is very high. CAPS is characterised by thromboses generating in two or more organs in a few days. That leads to infarction and necrosis of the affected tissues causing multiple organ failures [7].

Standard care for thrombotic APS is indefinite anticoagulation with a vitamin K antagonist [8]. There is currently insufficient evidence to recommend the routine use of direct oral anticoagulants (DOAC) in thrombotic APS [9].

The 13th Task Force recommendation for primary thromboprophylaxis in APS supports the use of aspirin [10]. A recent meta-analysis conducted on a total of 1208 asymptomatic patients with persistently positive aPL has shown that low-dose aspirin (LDA) is associated with significant risk reduction in arterial but not in venous thrombosis when compared to placebo [11]. Aspirin with low molecular weight or unfractionated heparin may reduce the incidence of pregnancy loss in obstetric APS [12]. Aspirin alone is advised for treating patients with aPL-associated stroke or acute myocardial infarction [13].

Treatment regimens of APS further include hydroxychloroquine, statins, B-cell inhibitors, complement inhibitors, blocking of aPL/B2 GPI receptors on target cells and tissue factor inhibitors [14].

A combined therapy of anticoagulation, glucocorticoids, plasma exchange and intravenous immunoglobulin (especially in the presence of infection) can be used in complicated cases of multiorgan failure due to thrombosis as in CAPS. Cyclophosphamide can also be used in CAPS in the presence of secondary autoimmune disease such as SLE [15]. Rituximab can also be used in refractory cases after failure or inability to take the above-mentioned combined therapies or in the presence of micro-angiopathic haemolytic anaemia [16].

However, the majority of aPL-positive patients do not have thrombosis. That is why the stereotypical treatment for APS patients should be avoided and stratification of the thrombotic

http://dx.doi.org/10.5772/intechopen.72509

risks is important as aPLs are prevalently observed in various diseases or elderly population. Current risk-stratification tools are largely limited to the antiphospholipid antibody profile and traditional thrombotic risk factors.

Novel biomarkers that correlate with disease activity and potentially provide insight into future clinical events include domain 1 specific anti-β2GPI antibodies, antibodies to other phospholipids, or phospholipid-protein complexes (such as antiphosphatidylserine/prothrombin antibodies (aPS/PT)), and functional/biological assays such as thrombin generation, complement activation, levels of circulating microparticles, and annexin A5 resistance [17].

Clinical risk scores (antiphospholipid score (aPL-S) and the Global Anti-phospholipid Syndrome Score [GAPSS]) may also have value in predicting clinical events [18].

2. Diagnosis of APS

Diagnosis of APS is based on the Sapporo criteria (proposed in 1999 and updated in 2006 after a conference in Sydney, Australia) [19].

These include at least one clinical and at least one laboratory manifestation of APS. Clinical criteria include objectively confirmed venous, arterial, or small vessel thrombosis, and/or obstetric morbidity including recurrent miscarriage, stillbirth, or intrauterine growth retardation.

The laboratory criteria require demonstration of a persistent presence of lupus anticoagulant (LA), anti-cardiolipin (ACA) or anti-2GPI antibody (IgG or IgM). Antiphospholipid antibody positivity can be stated if at least one of these antibodies could be detected twice, 12 weeks apart. LA is measured by the help of coagulation tests, while ACA and anti-β2glycoprotein 1 (aβ2GPI) are determined by means of ELISA. LA results are expressed as qualitative data and only strong positivity carries clinical significance. In case of ACA and aβ2GPI, antibody medium/high titres of IgM and/or IgG subtype have important clinical value (**Table 1**).

Clinical symptoms of APS include thrombosis in any blood vessel of any organ. Typically, thrombosis may recur and can present both in arteries and in veins. Anti-phospholipid antibodies represent the strongest thrombophiliac factors, mainly LA.

Although thrombosis due to APS does not differ from thrombosis caused by any other factors, some other symptoms and signs may accompany to the elevated blood clotting: for example, if a patient presents with thrombosis and also has livedo reticularis, it is very likely that thrombosis is a manifestation of APS.

Besides, there are only a few situations when arterious and venous thrombosis present on the same patient. This and the recurrence of the thrombotic event is very likely refers to APS.

There are the so-called "non-criteria" clinical features of APS, such as livedo reticularis, cardiac valve disease, haematological manifestations (thrombocytopenia and haemolytic anaemia), nephropathy and neurological manifestations (migraine, chorea and epilepsy).

Non-criteria manifestations mean that the presence of these characteristic features of the disease is not a requisite of the diagnosis, or with other words, they are not the *sine qua non* of the diagnosis.

Vascular thrombosis	≥1 clinical episode of arterial, venous or small vessel thrombosis. Thrombosis must be objectively confirmed. For histopathological confirmation, thrombosis must be present without inflammation of the vessel wall
Pregnancy morbidity	≥1 unexplained death of a morphologically normal foetus ≥10 weeks of gestation ≥1 premature delivery of a morphologically normal foetus <34 weeks of gestation because of: • severe preeclampsia or eclampsia defined according to standard definition; • recognised features of placental insufficiency ≥3 unexplained consecutive miscarriages <10 weeks of gestation, with maternal and paternal factors (anatomic, hormonal or chromosomal abnormalities) excluded
Laboratory criteria	Presence of antiphospholipid antibodies (aPLs), on two or more occasions at least 12 weeks apart and no more than 5 years prior to clinical manifestations, as demonstrated by ≥1 of the following: • Lupus anticoagulant; • Medium to high-titre (>40 GPL or MPL, or >99th percentile) anticardiolipin IgG or IgM; • Anti-β2 glycoprotein-I (anti-β2GPI) IgG or IgM >99th percentile

Table 1. Revised classification criteria for antiphospholipid syndrome [19].

Thrombocytopenia is the most relevant non-criteria manifestation of APS.

However, despite the pro-thrombotic nature of APS, thrombocytopenia is one of the most common non-criteria findings of the disease. Recently, thrombocytopenia is proposed to be a diagnostic clinical criterion of APS.

In case of OAPS several disease processes may occur in the placentae of women with antiphospholipid syndrome due to the antiphospholipid autoantibodies, not only thrombosis and infarction, but also inflammatory events, mediated by cytokine release, complement activation, angiogenic imbalance and activation of immune cells [20].

3. Epidemiology of APS

Presence of aPL Abs per se does not guarantee a patient will develop APS as only 8.1% of patients with aPL antibodies without a history of clinical thrombosis developed thrombosis during a 5-year follow-up period, suggesting that a patient needs an additional insult to develop the clinical disease [21, 22]. The prevalence of the antibodies increases with age [23].

Forty percent of patients with APS have SLE. The prevalence of ACA in SLE is from 12 to 30%, and LA is found in 5–34%. From the patients with SLE and aPL antibodies 50–70% progress to APS.

The incidence of the APS is around five new cases per 100,000 persons per year, and the prevalence is around 40–50 cases per 100,000 persons [24].

The aPLs are positive in approximately 13% of patients with stroke, 11% with myocardial infarction, 9.5% of patients with deep vein thrombosis and 6% of patients with pregnancy morbidity [16]. These data can underline the significance of APS.

According to another study, patients with cerebrovascular events who are less than 50 years old have shown 17.4% prevalence of positive aPL with five times increase in the risk of ischaemic stroke [25].

Thrombocytopenia is the most common non-criteria hematologic manifestation of APS. It has been reported with prevalence between 30 and 46% among APS patients [26].

There is a difference between primary and secondary APS patients in respect of the frequency of thrombocytopenia: in Euro-Phospholipid project, the frequency of thrombocytopenia in patients with PAPS was 21%, while it was 41.9% in patients with secondary APS [27].

4. Role of platelets in APS

Platelets play a key role in APS-related thrombosis due to the presence of multiple receptors that can interact with anti-β2-GPI antibodies (especially apolipoprotein E receptor 2′ (apoER2′) and glycoprotein Ibα (GPIbα)) with consequent release of different pro-coagulant mediators such as thromboxane B2, platelet factor 4 (PF4) and platelet factor 4 variant (CXCL4L1) [28].

In case of APS, thrombosis results from a hypercoagulable state caused by activation of endothelial cells, monocytes and platelets. It has been demonstrated that platelets are required for enhanced activation of the endothelium and fibrin generation by the anti-β2GP1 autoantibody/β2GP1 complex. Thus, the first event is the activation of thrombocytes, endothelial cells are activated indirectly [29].

Platelet activation, a major contributing factor of arterial thrombosis in APS, might play a role in APS-related thrombosis in at least two ways:

First, due to the presence of multiple receptors that can interact with antibodies, platelets can facilitate the dimerisation of β2-GPI enhancing the coagulation response.

Second, platelets provide a surface for coagulation reactions [30].

The role of thrombocytes in the pathogenesis of APS is supported by the fact that circulating platelet- and endothelial-derived microparticle level are elevated in patients with primary APS [31].

Mouse models of APS have shown that platelets are the first target for circulating anti-β2-GPI-β2-GPI complexes, and the enhancement of endothelium activation is also platelet thrombus-dependent [29].

5. About thrombocytopenia in general

The normal value of platelet count is between 150 and 300 $\times$ 10^9/L. Platelet number between 100 and 150 $\times$ 10^9/L is considered as normal in some studies. That may be the cause of some controversial research data. Decreased thrombocyte number might be present because of

Increased platelet activation and destruction	
Immune-mediated (aPL-related, secondary ITP)	
Thrombotic microangiopathy (CAPS, HELLP syndrome, HUS, TTP)	
Drug-induced (e.g., heparin)	
Decreased platelet production	
Haemophagocytic syndrome	
Bone marrow necrosis	
Increased platelet pooling	
Pseudothrombocytopenia	

CAPS: catastrophic antiphospholipid syndrome; HELLP: hemolysis, elevated liver enzymes, and low platelet count; aHUS: atypical hemolytic uremic syndrome; TTP: thrombotic thrombocytopenic purpura.

Table 2. Mechanisms of thrombocytopenia in antiphospholipid antibody (aPL)-positive patients [34].

several reasons. The two main categories are the decreased thrombopoiesis in the bone marrow and the increased destruction of platelets in the peripheral blood [32].

Consequences depend on the degree of thrombocytopenia: under 20×10^9/L it is considered severe, between 20 and 50×10^9/L moderate and above 50×10^9/L mild thrombocytopenia [33].

It is not only the number but also the thrombocyte function has a great importance in respect of consequences of thrombocytopenia: even a few thrombocytes can provide a satisfactory performance if the underlying disease does not diminish thrombocyte function. For example, in case of acute leukaemia patient may have bleeding even with a higher platelet number than that patient with immune thrombocytopenic purpura (ITP) who will be fine with a much lower thrombocyte count.

In case of the so-called consumptive thrombocytopenia, the basic phenomenon is the activation of platelets. Activation leads to thrombosis generation, factors of blood coagulation such as platelets are utilised and the thrombocyte number will decrease. As a secondary process bleeding occurs (**Table 2**).

6. Thrombocytopenia in APS

Thrombocytopenia is frequently found in patients with the APS and is usually mild (70–120 $\times 10^9$/L) and benign, with no intervention required. In a few cases it can be severe and aggressive treatment may be required. Low platelet counts usually appear associated with other APS manifestations, but sometimes it may be the only sign of APS [35].

The same working group has compared the frequency of thrombocytopenia in different subgroups of APS. They found no differences in the occurrence of low platelet number in patients with primary or secondary APS [35].

Thrombocytopenia is a frequent phenomenon of SLE. Increased concentrations of aPL antibodies have been found to be common in patients not only with SLE, but also with immune thrombocytopenic purpura (ITP). No clinical significance or role in mechanisms of thrombocytopenia of aPL antibodies was found [36]. In an earlier study, about 30% of ITP patients had a positive aCL test at the time of diagnosis [37]. In case of Evans syndrome (thrombocytopenia and haemolytic anaemia) aPL autoantibodies are also frequently present.

7. Pathogenesis of thrombocytopenia in APS

The pathogenesis of thrombocytopenia related to aPL antibodies is still unclear. It is possibly caused by direct binding of anti-β2-GPI antibodies or anti-β2-GPI-β2-GPI complexes on activated platelets and promotes their aggregation and thrombus formation, so thrombocytopenia is a consequence of consumption of platelets.

On the other hand, thrombocytopenia in APS may be due to immune-mediated clearance of platelets, as in case of ITP [38].

8. Characterisation of thrombocytopenia in APS

Thrombocytopenia in APS is usually mild (70–120 $\times$ 10^9/L) and does not require clinical intervention. In most of the cases, the main significance of thrombocytopenia is that it can be a sign, and when noticed it, the presence of aPL antibodies can be found. Severe thrombocytopenia (platelet count <50 $\times$ 10^9/L) may be seen in 5–10% of patients [37].

9. Clinical significance of thrombocytopenia in APS

Interestingly, the presence of thrombocytopenia in patients with APS is not typically associated with haemorrhagic complications; rather it can trigger thrombotic events. Even more, it has been proven that the more severe the thrombocytopenia, the higher the probability of future thrombosis.

In a retrospective study 138 patients were enrolled with positive aPL without fulfilling clinical criteria for APS, after a mean follow-up of 146 $\pm$ 60.3 months, 29.4% with thrombocytopenia developed thrombosis. They concluded that aPL-positive patients who develop thrombocytopenia have a potential risk of developing thrombosis [39].

Platelet activation plays an essential role in the development of atherosclerosis. In case of arterial thrombosis, the role of platelets is also essential. Continuous platelet activation in patients with APS may be involved, among other factors, in accelerated atherosclerosis. Moreover, atherosclerosis and its thrombotic complications may be mediated by local secretion of molecular effectors embedded or packed into microvesicles from the platelet surface [40].

A fundamental role of platelets and platelet activation in the process of thrombosis generation of APS patients has been supported by several data. These data suggest that aPL antibodies do not interact with circulating platelets in these patients. Instead, anti-β2-GPI-β2-GPI complexes bind exclusively to the platelet thrombus and not to the endothelium, a phenomenon leading to the amplification of platelet activation [29]. A possible explanation might be that aCL antibodies are able to bind the lipid component of platelet membrane only after platelet activation. In fact, major binding targets are the anionic phospholipids phosphatidyl-serine (PS), phosphatidylinositol (PI), and phosphatidyl-ethanolamine (PE), located in the inner surface of the platelet lipid membrane that becomes exposed and accessible to anti-β2-GPI antibodies after platelet activation.

10. Thrombocytopenia and risk stratification

Among aPL-positive patients, those with a low platelet count developed thrombosis more frequently than those without. Among aPL-negative patients, no difference was found in the predictive value of thrombosis regardless of platelet count [29].

11. Mean platelet volume (MPV) in APS

Beside thrombocytopenia, MCV alterations may have significant importance in APS. Though conformation of data is still lacking, there are evidences that platelets with increased MPV are more active than smaller platelets, with a greater pro-thrombotic potential because of higher levels of intracellular TXA2 and an increased pro-coagulant surface [41]. MPV is largely regarded as a useful surrogate marker of platelet activation [42].

MPV was found to be significantly higher in APS patients, especially in triple positive patients, as compared to controls. Moreover, the level of MPV above 7.4 fl was found to be an independent predictor of thrombosis recurrence in patients with APS [43].

12. Differential diagnosis of thrombocytopenia in APS

Pseudo-thrombocytopenia should be excluded. Presence of fragmentocytes can refer to TTP. The observation of the characteristic "pentad" (fever, microangiopathic anaemia, thrombocytopenia, neurologic abnormalities and renal involvement) may strengthen the diagnosis.

Bone marrow examination can show out malignant haematological diseases such as multiple myeloma, or different kind of leukaemia, when there is no place for normal thrombopoiesis.

In case of myelodysplastic syndrome (MDS), there are dysplastic features of the cells of megakaryocytic cell line and also morphological abnormalities of thrombocytes can be observed in the peripheral smear.

Haemolytic anaemia is indicative of secondary APS due to SLE, or Evans syndrome. Otherwise, in case of SLE, not only haemolytic anaemia and thrombocytopenia may be found, but also aPL antibodies, without any clinical symptoms of APS. Other clinical symptoms of the systemic autoimmune disease or a history of thrombosis can help to differentiate, but it is not always an easy task.

Immune-thrombocytopenic purpura (ITP) is the most frequent cause of "megakaryocytic" thrombocytopenia. It is typically an exclusion diagnosis: when we cannot find any other reason of decreased platelet number, and there are megakaryocytes in the bone marrow we consider ITP.

Thrombocytopenia is often experienced in pregnancy, affecting up to 10% of all pregnancies [44]. The causes of pregnancy-specific thrombocytopenia are gestational thrombocytopenia, pre-eclampsia, HELLP syndrome and acute fatty liver of pregnancy.

The most common cause of thrombocytopenia in pregnancy is gestational thrombocytopenia (75% of all cases) [45]. It may be difficult to differentiate from ITP, which also presents frequently during pregnancy, mainly in the first and second trimester. However, gestational thrombocytopenia generally causes mild thrombocytopenia, usually $>70 \times 10^9$/L, from the mid-second or third trimester, and is not related to adverse events for the mother and new-born. In some cases, pregnancy might lead to worsening of thrombocytopenia in patients with ITP [46]. This may be caused by the effects of the hormonal milieu of pregnancy on the reticuloendothelial system.

Thrombocytopenia is usually mild during pregnancy and is caused mainly by haemodilution. However, ITP, or SLE, even APS can start during pregnancy. Therefore complete examination of the patient, thorough laboratory checking, detailed medical history and careful follow-up is crucial.

13. How to treat thrombocytopenia in APS?

The first task is to exclude concomitant SLE, or ITP, and ascertain whether thrombocytopenia refers to an increased activation of the coagulation system or an elevated tendency of bleeding. If it has been proven that thrombocytopenia is the manifestation of APS, it might have great importance: it can predict later thrombosis.

As thrombocytopenia is usually mild and if it predicts later thrombosis, usually APS can be treated by standard therapy. Patients can be given platelet aggregation inhibitors and/or anticoagulant therapy. Anti-thrombotic treatment should be stopped only in case of severe thrombocytopenia or bleeding [34].

In the presence of severe thrombocytopenia, rituximab represents a unique drug which can balance the effect of bleeding and thrombosis. By reducing the production of autoantibodies, rituximab can simultaneously raise the platelets and reduce the chance of thrombosis. Rituximab can supersede splenectomy as a second-line therapy in this group of patients [47].

In case of SLE-associated APS, when severe thrombocytopenia is generated by disease activation SLE should be treated with high-dose glucocorticoids, IVIG, immunosuppressive agents and plasma exchange [48, 49].

CAPS is a life-threatening disease that requires very aggressive treatment. The treatment strategy is based on the combination of anticoagulation, glucocorticoids, plasma exchange and/or intravenous immunoglobulin, the so-called triple therapy. In refractory cases or in those with initial life-threatening situation, rituximab may be an effective option [15]. Recently, some cases of CAPS have been effectively treated with the addition of eculizumab to the triple therapy [50].

In case of pregnancy-associated APS, the health of the mother is considered always the more important. If there is a life-threatening situation, the pregnancy must be terminated. Pregnancy itself represents a higher thrombotic risk, so careful anticoagulation is extremely important. On the other hand, bleeding during delivery also should be avoided.

14. Conclusion

Thrombocytopenia may be a symptom of APS. Paradoxically, it refers to an elevated thrombotic tendency, not bleeding risk. The causes of decreased platelet number are complex: antiphospholipid antibodies that bind to platelets activate them and induce thrombosis. Thrombocytes are consumed during this process. On the other hand, thrombocytopenia is the consequence of destruction by immune mechanisms, like in the case of ITP. Sometimes, it might be the only sign of APS.

Diagnosis is not easy; other causes of thrombocytopenia must be excluded by careful examinations.

Thrombocytopenia in APS is usually mild and *per se* does not require any treatment. Patients with or without thrombocytopenia require anticoagulant medication in case of venous thrombotic event while low-dose aspirin or clopidogrel is recommended after arterial thrombosis. For OAPS, the combination of anticoagulant and thrombocyte aggregation inhibitor therapy is advised. CAPS is a life-threatening disease with a rapid progression of multiorgan failure. Even application of high-dose corticosteroids, plasma exchange, intravenous immunoglobulin and complement inhibitor agent mortality is very high.

Abbreviations

APS	antiphospholipid syndrome
aPL	antiphospholipid antibody
aβ2GPI	anti-β2 glycoprotein 1
ACA	anti-cardiolipin antibody
CAPS	catastrophic antiphospholipid syndrome
DOAC	direct oral anticoagulants
ITP	immune thrombocytopenic purpura
LA	lupus anticoagulant
MDS	myelodysplastic syndrome
OAPS	obstetric antiphospholipid syndrome
SLE	systemic lupus erythematodes
TTP	thrombotic thrombocytopenic purpura

http://dx.doi.org/10.5772/intechopen.72509

Conflict of interest

There is no conflict of interest.

Author details

Klara Gadó[1]* and Gyula Domján[2]

*Address all correspondence to: gadok@freemail.hu

1 Faculty of Health Sciences, Department of Clinical Studies, Semmelweis University of Medicine, Budapest, Hungary

2 Faculty of Medicine, 1st Department of Medicine, Semmelweis University of Medicine, Budapest, Hungary

References

[1] Hughes GRV. Thrombosis, abortion, cerebral disease and lupus anticoagulant. BMJ. 1983;**287**:1088-1089

[2] Pengo V, Tripodi A, Reber G, et al. Update of the guidelines for lupus anticoagulant detection: Subcommittee on Lupus Anticoagulant/antiphospholipid Antibody of the Scientific and Standardisation Committee of the International Society on Thrombosis and Haemostasis. Journal of Thrombosis and Haemostasis. 2009;**7**(10):1737-1740

[3] Petri M. Hughes syndrome: Antiphospholipid syndrome. In: Khamashta MA, editor. Hughes Syndrome Vol. 1. 2nd ed. London: Springer-Verlag London Ltd; 2006. pp. 22-28

[4] Hughes GR, Khamashta MA. The antiphospholipid syndrome. Journal of the Royal College of Physicians of London. 1994;**28**(4):301-304

[5] Camarena Cabrera DM, Rodriguez-Jaimes C, Acevedo-Gallegos S, Gallardo-Gaona JM, Velazquez-Torres B, Ramírez-Calvo JA. Controversies concerning the antiphospholipid syndrome in obstetrics. Clinical Rheumatology. 2017;**13**(1):30-36

[6] Levy RA, Dos Santos FC, de Jesús GR, de Jesús NR. Antiphospholipid antibodies and Antiphospholipid syndrome during pregnancy: Diagnostic concepts. Frontiers in Immunology. 2015;**6**:205

[7] Kazzaz NM, McCune WJ, Knight JS. Treatment of catastrophic antiphospholipid syndrome. Current Opinion in Rheumatology. 2016 May;**28**(3):218-227

[8] Pengo V, Ruiz-Irastorza G, Denas G, et al. High intensity anticoagulation in the prevention of the recurrence of arterial thrombosis in antiphospholipid syndrome: 'PROS' and 'CONS'. Autoimmunity Reviews. 2012;**11**:577-580

[9] Joshi A, Hong J, Siva C. Recurrent thrombosis in patients with antiphospholipid syndrome receiving newer oral anticoagulants: A case report and review of literature. Clinical Medicine & Research. 2017;**15**(1–2):41-44

[10] Arnaud L, Mathian A, Ruffatti A, Erkan D, Tektonidou M, Cervera R, Forastiero R, Pengo V, Lambert M, Martinez-Zamora MA, Balasch J, Zuily S, Wahl D, Amoura Z. Efficacy of aspirin for the primary prevention of thrombosis in patients with antiphospholipid antibodies: An international and collaborative meta-analysis. Autoimmunity Reviews. 2014;**13**(3):281-291

[11] Derksen RH, de Groot PG. Towards evidence-based treatment of thrombotic antiphospholipid syndrome. Lupus. 2010;**19**(4):470-474

[12] Hoppe B, Burmester GR, Dörner T. Heparin or aspirin or both in the treatment of recurrent abortions in women with antiphospholipid antibody (syndrome). Current Opinion in Rheumatology. 2011;**23**(3):299-304

[13] Okuma H, Kitagawa Y, Yasuda T, Tokuoka K, Takagi S. Comparison between single antiplatelet therapy and combination of antiplatelet and anticoagulation therapy for secondary prevention in ischemic stroke patients with antiphospholipid syndrome. International Journal of Medical Sciences. 2009;**7**(1):15-18

[14] Al Marzooqi A, Leone A, Al Saleh J, Khamashta M. Current status and future prospects for the treatment of antiphospholipid syndrome. Expert Review of Clinical Immunology. 2016;**12**(9):927-935

[15] Espinosa G, Rodríguez-Pintó I, Cervera R. Catastrophic antiphospholipid syndrome: An update. Panminerva Medica. 2017;**59**(3):254-268

[16] Merashli M, Noureldine MH, Uthman I, Khamashta M. Antiphospholipid syndrome: An update. European Journal of Clinical Investigation. 2015;**45**(6):653-662. DOI: 10.1111/eci.12449

[17] Chaturvedi S, McCrae KR. Clinical risk assessment in the antiphospholipid syndrome: Current landscape and emerging biomarkers. Current Rheumatology Reports. 2017;**19**(7):43

[18] Oku K, Amengual O, Yasuda S, Atsumi T. How to identify high-risk APS patients: Clinical utility and predictive values of validated scores. Current Rheumatology Reports. 2017;**19**(8):51

[19] Miyakis S, Lockshin MD, Atsumi T, et al. International consensus statement on an update of the classification criteria for definite antiphospholipid syndrome (APS). Journal of Thrombosis and Haemostasis. 2006;**4**:295-306

[20] Mulla MJ, Brosens JJ, Chamley LW, Giles I, Pericleous C, Rahman A, et al. Antiphospholipid antibodies induce a pro-inflammatory response in first trimester trophoblast via the TLR4/ MyD88pathway. American Journal of Reproductive Immunology. 2009;**62**:96-111

[21] Mustonen P, Lehtonen KV, Javela K, Puurunen M. Persistent antiphospholipid antibody (aPL) in asymptomatic carriers as a risk factor for future thrombotic events: A nationwide prospective study. Lupus. 2014;**23**(14):1468-1476

[22] Ruffatti A, Del Ross T, Ciprian M, Nuzzo M, Rampudda M, Bertero MT, Bergia R, Caramaschi P, Biasi D, Capsoni F, Montaguti L, Ruffini R, Brucato A, Picillo U, Fanelli V,

Riccieri V, Piccoli A, Valesini G, Doria A, Meroni PL, Tincani A. Risk factors for a first thrombotic event in antiphospholipid antibody carriers. A multicentre, retrospective follow-up study. Annals of the Rheumatic Diseases. 2009;**68**(3):397-399

[23] Manukyan D, Rossmann H, Schulz A, Zeller T, Pfeiffer N, Binder H, Münzel T, Beutel ME, Müller-Calleja N, Wild PS, Lackner KJ. Distribution of antiphospholipid antibodies in a large population-based German cohort. Clinical Chemistry and Laboratory Medicine. 2016;**54**(10):1663-1670

[24] Neville C, Rauch J, Kassis J, Chang ER, Joseph L, Le Comte M, Fortin PR. Thromboembolic risk in patients with high titre anticardiolipin and multiple antiphospholipid antibodies. Thrombosis and Haemostasis. 2003;**90**(1):108-115

[25] Sciascia S, Sanna G, Khamashta MA, Cuadrado MJ, Erkan D, Andreoli L, et al. The estimated frequency of antiphospholipid antibodies in young adults with cerebrovascular events: A systematic review. Annals of the Rheumatic Diseases. 2015;**74**(11):2028-2033

[26] Sciascia S, Amigo MC, Roccatello D, Khamashta M. Diagnosing antiphospholipid syndrome: 'extra-criteria' manifestations and technical advances. Nature Reviews Rheumatology. 2017;**13**(9):548-560

[27] Cervera R, Piette JC, Font J, et al. Antiphospholipid syndrome: Clinical and immunologic manifestations and patterns of disease expression in a cohort of 1,000 patients. Arthritis and Rheumatism. 2002;**46**(4):1019-1027

[28] Baroni G, Banzato A, Bison E, Denas G, Zoppellaro G, Pengo V. The role of platelets in antiphospholipid syndrome. Platelets. 2017;**7**:1-5

[29] Proulle V, Furie RA, Merrill-Skoloff G, Furie BC, Furie B. Platelets are required for enhanced activation of the endothelium and fibrinogen in a mouse thrombosis model of APS. Blood. 2014;**124**(4):611-622

[30] Vlachoyiannopoulos PG, Routsias JG. A novel mechanism of thrombosis in antiphospholipid antibody syndrome. Journal of Autoimmunity. 2010;**35**(3):248-255

[31] Breen KA, Sanchez K, Kirkman N, Seed PT, Parmar K, Moore GW, Hunt BJ. Endothelial and platelet microparticles in patients with antiphospholipid antibodies. Thrombosis Research. 2015;**135**(2):368-374

[32] Ali N, Auerbach HE. New-onset acute thrombocytopenia in hospitalized patients: Pathophysiology and diagnostic approach. Journal of Community Hospital Internal Medicine Perspectives. 2017;**7**(3):157-167

[33] Buckley MF, James JW, Brown DE, et al. A novel approach to the assessment of variations in the human platelet count. Thrombosis and Haemostasis. 2000;**83**(3):480-484

[34] Artim-Esen B, Diz-Küçükkaya R, İnanç M. The significance and management of thrombocytopenia in antiphospholipid syndrome. Current Rheumatology Reports. 2015;**17**(3):14

[35] Cuadrado MJ, Mujic F, Muñoz E, Khamashta MA, Hughes GRV. Thrombocytopenia in the antiphospholipid syndrome. Annals of the Rheumatic Diseases. 1997;**56**:194-196

[36] Stasi R, Stipa E, Masi M, Oliva F, Sciarra A, Perroti A, et al. Prevalence and clinical significance of elevated antiphospholipid antibodies in patients with idiopathic thrombocytopenic purpura. Blood. 1994;**84**:4203-4208

[37] Harris EN, Gharavi AE, Hedge U, Derue G, Morgan SH, Englert H, et al. Anticardiolipin antibodies in autoimmune thrombocytopenic purpura. British Journal of Haematology. 1985;**59**:231-234

[38] Abreu MM, Danowski A, Wahl DG, Amigo MC, Tektonidou M, Pacheco MS, Fleming N, Domingues V, Sciascia S, Lyra JO, Petri M, Khamashta M, Levy RA. The relevance of "non-criteria" clinical manifestations of antiphospholipid syndrome: 14th International Congress on Antiphospholipid Antibodies Technical Task Force Report on Antiphospholipid Syndrome Clinical Features. Autoimmunity Reviews. 2015;**14**(5):401-414

[39] Demetrio Pablo R, Muñoz P, López-Hoyos M, Calvo V, Riancho L, Martínez-Taboada VM. Thrombocytopenia as a thrombotic risk factor in patients with antiphospholipid antibodies without disease criteria. Medicina Clínica (Barcelona). 2017;**148**(9):394-400

[40] Palomo I, Toro C, Alarcon M. The role of platelets in the pathophysiology of atherosclerosis (review). Molecular Medicine Reports. 2008;**1**(2):179-184

[41] Kamath S, Blann AD, Lip GY. Platelet activation: Assessment and quantification. European Heart Journal. 2001;**22**(17):1561-1571

[42] Korkmaz S, Uslu AU, Sahin S, Senel S, Sencan MI. There a link between mean platelet volume and thrombotic events in antiphospholipid syndrome? Platelets. 2014;**25**(5):343-347

[43] Rupa-Matysek J, Gil L, Wojtasinska E, Ciepluch K, Lewandowska M, Komarnicki M. The relationship between mean platelet volume and thrombosis recurrence in patients diagnosed with antiphospholipid syndrome. Rheumatology International. 2014;**34**(11):1599-1605

[44] Myers B. Diagnosis and management of maternal thrombocytopenia in pregnancy. British Journal of Haematology. 2012;**158**(1):3-15

[45] Gernsheimer T, James AH, Stasi R. How I treat thrombocytopenia in pregnancy. Blood. 2013;**121**(1):38-47

[46] Sun D, Shehata N, Ye XY, Gregorovich S, De France B, Arnold DM, Shah PS, Malinowski AK. Corticosteroids compared with intravenous immunoglobulin for the treatment of immune thrombocytopenia in pregnancy. Blood. 2016;**128**(10):1329-1335

[47] Gamoudi D, Cutajar M, Gamoudi N, Camilleri DJ, Gatt A. Achieving a satisfactory clinical and biochemical response in antiphospholipid syndrome and severe thrombocytopenia with rituximab: Two case reports. Clinical Case Reports. 2017;**5**(6):845-848

[48] Pons-Estel GJ, Andreoli L, Scanzi F, Cervera R, Tincani A. The antiphospholipid syndrome in patients with systemic lupus erythematosus. Journal of Autoimmunity. 2017;**76**:10-20

[49] Martirosyan A, Petrek M, Kishore A, Manukyan G. Immunomodulatory effects of therapeutic plasma exchange on monocytes in antiphospholipid syndrome. Experimental and Therapeutic Medicine. 2016;**12**(2):1189-1195

[50] Gustavsen A, Skattum L, Bergseth G, Lorentzen B, Floisand Y, Bosnes V, Mollnes TE, Barratt-Due A. Effect on mother and child of eculizumab given before caesarean section in a patient with severe antiphospholipid syndrome: A case report. Medicine (Baltimore). 2017;**96**(11):e6338

Chapter 5

Interferon-Induced Thrombotic Microangiopathy

Ajay Kundra, Mirela Andrei and Jen Chin Wang

Additional information is available at the end of the chapter

http://dx.doi.org/10.5772/intechopen.74226

Abstract

Interferon (IFN) is an effective therapy for multiple disorders. An infrequently reported side effect is thrombotic microangiopathy (TMA): thrombotic thrombocytopenic purpura (TTP) and hemolytic uremic syndrome (HUS). We published the first comprehensive review analyzing this association with the following observations: (1) there was a higher incidence of IFN-induced TMA in myeloproliferative disorders (chronic myelogenous leukemia (CML)) than that in nonmalignant disorders (multiple sclerosis (MS), chronic hepatitis C virus infection (HCV)); (2) mean age at diagnosis was 47 years; (3) there was rare association with hairy cell leukemia (HCL), Sezary syndrome (one case each) and no cases reported for polycythemia vera (PV); (4) sex distribution was balanced (exception of higher prevalence in females for MS); (5) TMA was insidious in onset with long incubation periods (average treatment duration 40.4 months); (6) comparative analysis of mean time (months) to onset of TMA ensuing cumulative IFN exposure was: MS 68.6 vs. CML 35.5 vs. HCV 30.4; (7) confirmed TTP (low ADAMTS 13 levels) was associated with the presence of an inhibitor; (8) outcome analysis revealed complete remission in 27 (40%), persistent chronic kidney disease in 28 (42%) and fatality in 12 patients (18%); (9) corticosteroids, plasma exchange (PEX) and rituximab are effective therapies.

Keywords: thrombocytopenia, interferon, thrombotic microangiopathy (TMA), thrombotic thrombocytopenia purpura (TTP), myeloproliferative disorder, HCV

1. Introduction

Thrombocytopenia is a common side effect of IFN treatment. TMA is a distinct clinical entity with potentially fatal consequences without precise and expeditious intervention. Classic clinical presentation includes a triad of anemia, thrombocytopenia, and evidence of microangiopathic hemolysis on the peripheral blood smear. The quintessential pathologic feature is the development of microvascular thrombi affecting small or larger vessels with variable organ involvement. TMA, including TTP, is associated with a broad spectrum of conditions such as hemolytic uremic syndrome (HUS), disseminated intravascular coagulation (DIC), malignant hypertension, infections, autoimmune disorders and drugs. Irrespective of etiology, endothelial damage is the fundamental process and is instrumental in the generation of intravascular microthrombi [1]. Furthermore, TTP is characterized by decreased ADAMTS-13 levels, with most patients having severe deficiency (<10%). There was no prior precedent of a comprehensive review exploring IFN-associated TMA. We performed a PubMed search of all articles published between January 1993 and July 2016, focusing on interferon-induced TMA cross-referenced with the following terms: thrombotic thrombocytopenic purpura (TTP), IFN and thrombocytopenia, thrombotic microangiopathies, ADAMTS-13, autoimmune disease and IFN, interferon and hepatitis C, IFN and CML, IFN and multiple myeloma, IFN and renal cell cancer, IFN and polycythemia vera, IFN and lymphoma. Our analysis of this data was published in an exclusive review [2] with results outlined in the following sections.

2. Results

2.1. Age

Majority of patients were between 40 and 60 years of age. Mean ± SE was 47 (95% CI, 44–50). There was no correlation between age and duration of interferon treatment (**Figure 1**). For comparison of older (≥60 years) to younger (<60 years) patients with regard to the duration of IFN treatment, Mann Whitney U test was used; median and interquartile range (in months)

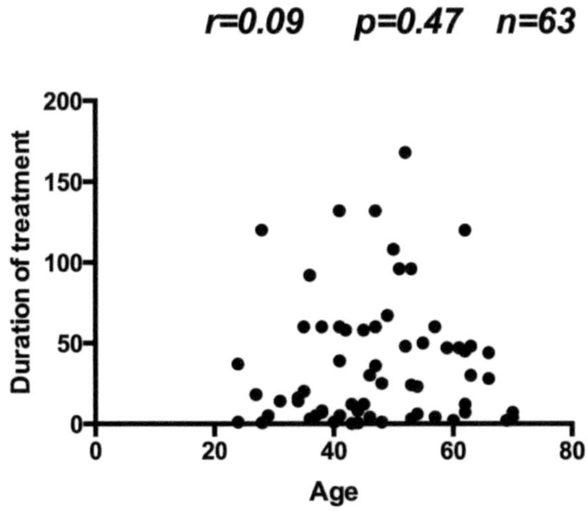

Figure 1. Correlation of age to duration of interferon (IFN) treatment before developing TMA. Sixty-eight patients including 29 CML, 20 MS, 17 Hepatitis C, 1 hairy cell leukemia, and 1 Sezary syndrome were studied. Correlation analysis using nonparametric Spearman's method was used to correlate age and duration of treatment (months). No significant correlation between age and duration of IFN usage was found.

http://dx.doi.org/10.5772/intechopen.74226

were (28, 5.5–46) and (23.50, 5–60) for older and younger age groups, respectively. Results were not statistically significant (**Figure 2**).

2.2. Sex

On cumulative data review, for the cases where information was available, sex distribution was balanced (30 male and 33 female patients). In subgroup analysis, patients with MS treated with IFNβ had a female predominance (12 out of 16; 75%). This may, however, just be reflective of higher prevalence of MS in women.

2.3. Associated clinical conditions

An aggregate of 68 cases reported from January 1993 to July 2016 was reviewed. The chronologic distribution of cases of IFN-induced TMA based on underlying diagnosis is shown in **Figure 3**. Incidence was highest in patients with CML followed by MS and HCV (29, 20 and 17, respectively) [3–44]. One case each was reported in patients with hairy cell leukemia (HCL) and Sezary syndrome [45, 46]. There have been no reports in patients with CML in the last 10 years correlating with the change in standard of care for the treatment of CML with tyrosine kinase inhibitors. There was no apparent difference in age distribution based on diagnosis. The cumulative duration of IFN exposure was highest in patients with MS treated with IFN β when compared to CML or HCV treated with IFN α: mean (months) ± SE: MS 68.6 (95% CI, 45.85–91.4), CML 35 (95% CI, 25.3–45.7) and HCV 12 (95% CI, 0.14–23.94). This was statistically significant (**Figure 4**) and is probably due to the difference in interferon type or different disease entity (IFNβ in MS vs. IFNα in CML and HCV).

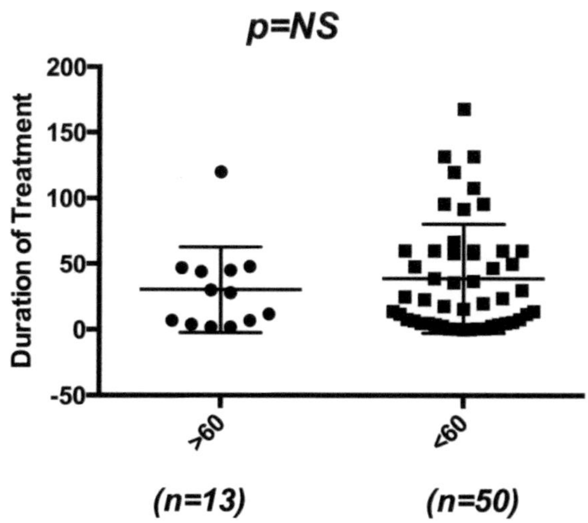

Figure 2. Comparison between older age (≥60) with younger age (<60) in relation to the duration of IFN usage. In order to compare older (≥60 years) to younger (<60 years) patients with regard to the duration of interferon treatment, Mann Whitney U test was used; median and interquartile range (in months) were (28, 5.5–46) and (23.50, 5–60) for older and younger age groups, respectively. No statistical significance was found.

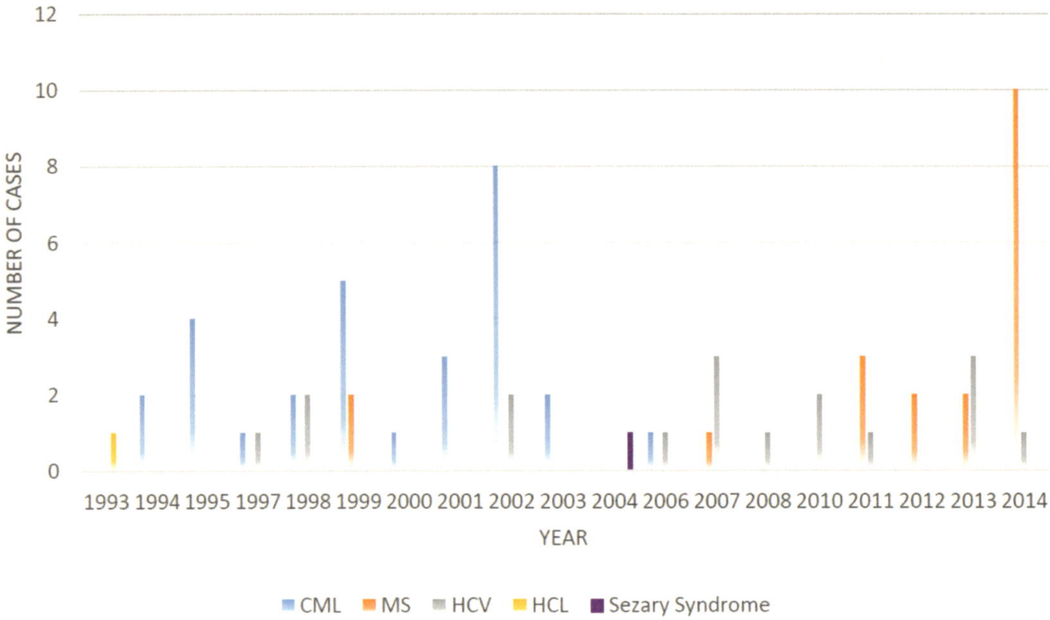

Figure 3. Incidence of reported cases of thrombotic microangiopathy by year and diagnosis: Results of incidence data analysis from the first reported case of IFN-induced TMA in 1993 to July 2016.

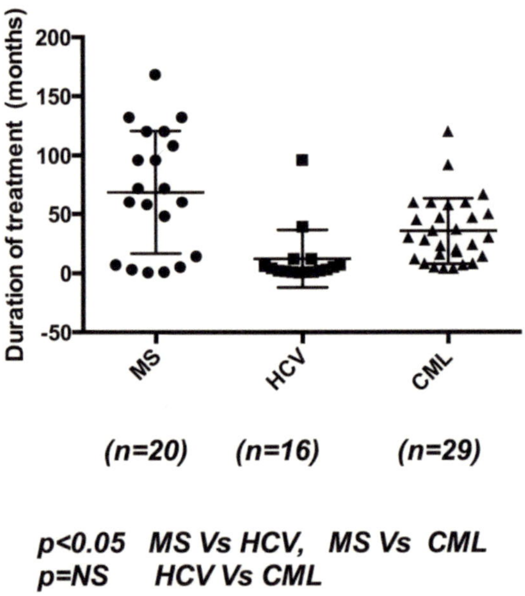

Figure 4. Comparison of cumulative IFN dose exposure prior to the onset of TMA in patients with CML, Hepatitis C, MS. Patients with MS treated with IFNβ showed longest duration of treatment exposure prior to the onset of TMA in comparison with patients with CML and hepatitis C treated with IFNα. Data were statistically significant.

Predominant clinical presentation was neurologic dysfunction, anemia, thrombocytopenia, and renal insufficiency. Platelet counts were analyzed for 50 patients where complete blood count (CBC) data were available. Sixteen patients were diagnosed with TTP based on clinical presentation, low ADAMTS13 level, renal biopsy or other evidence of TMA and the remaining as HUS, TTP-HUS or TMA. We grouped the latter for the purpose of our analysis as TMA unspecified. It appears that all patients with TTP presented with moderate-to-severe thrombocytopenia. In the group TMA unspecified, this was not a consistent finding (**Figure 5**). A significant number of patients were diagnosed as having TMA based on characteristic renal biopsy findings of microangiopathy. There were no other clearly discernible features that set these subgroups of patients apart.

2.4. Treatment and outcome

In our review of the 63 patients with available treatment data, 35 (56%) were treated with plasma exchange (PEX) with or without steroids, 12 (19%) were treated with steroids with or without plasma infusion, and 16 (25%) were treated by other means including IFN discontinuation or dose reduction, antihypertensive treatment, rituximab and hemodialysis. Of the 67 patients with available outcome data, 27 patients (40%) had complete response, 28 (42%) developed persistent CKD and 12 (18%) had a fatal outcome (**Figure 6**).

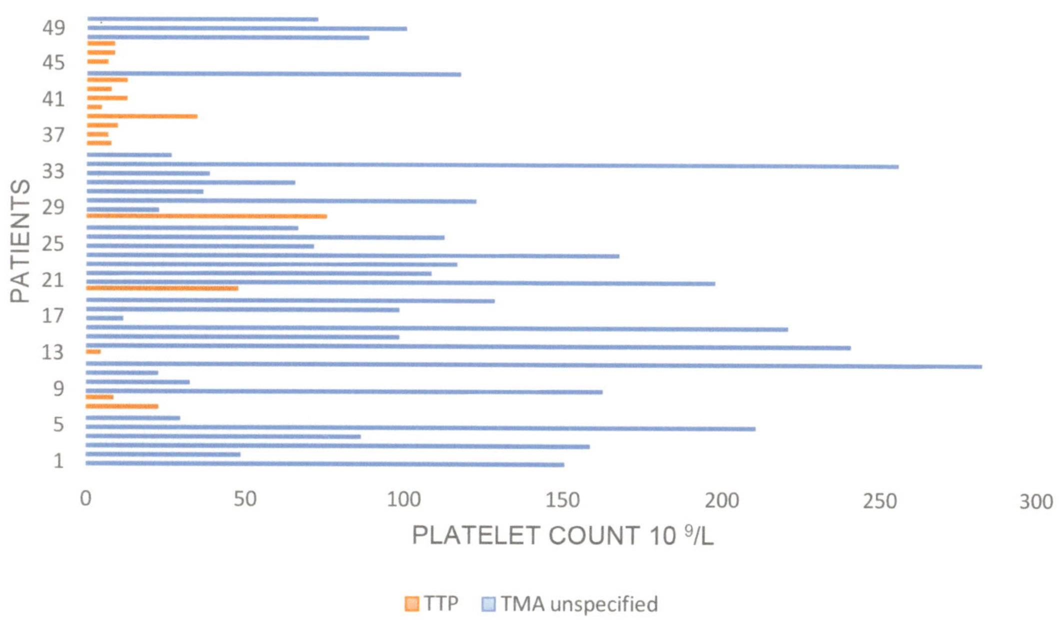

Figure 5. Platelet count trend at the time of diagnosis of TTP and TMA unspecified. Out of the 50 patients with available CBC data, 16 were diagnosed as TTP and rest as HUS, TTP-HUS or TMA. Data from the latter group of patients were pooled for the purpose of analysis as TMA unspecified. Patients with TTP presented consistently with moderate-to-severe thrombocytopenia, whereas there were wide fluctuations in platelet counts in patients with TMA unspecified.

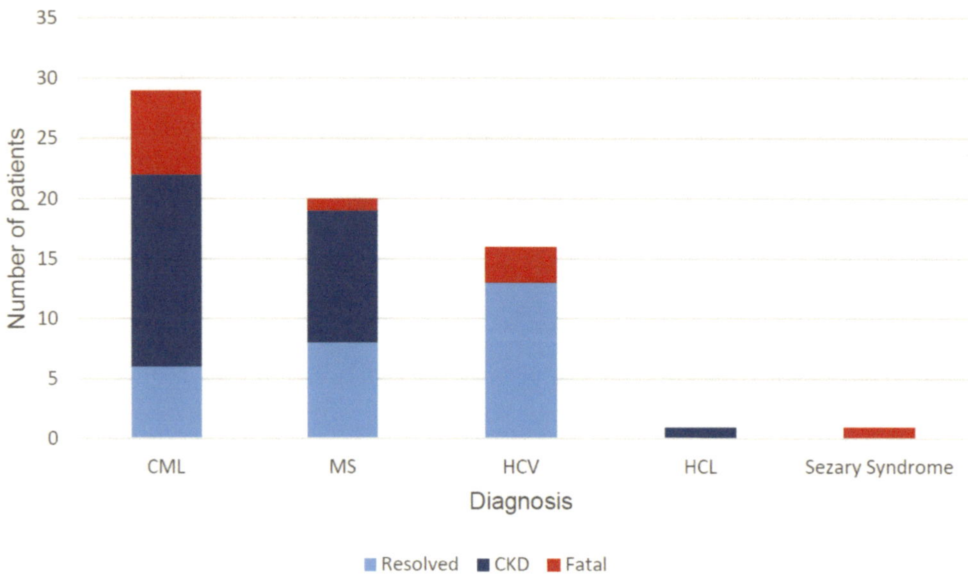

Figure 6. Outcome analysis data: Of the 67 patients with available outcome data, 27 patients (40%) had complete response, 28 (42%) developed persistent CKD and 12 (18%) died. Data were shown by underlying diagnosis.

2.5. Role of ADAMTS-13 inhibitor

There were eight cases of TTP where low ADAMTS 13 level was demonstrated, six of these also had ADAMTS 13 inhibitor. Notably, all patients with ADAMTS 13 inhibitor responded to PEX, steroids, and, in resistant cases, rituximab and vincristine. These results imply that IFN-induced TTP is probably an immune-mediated phenomenon with immune suppression being a key therapeutic intervention. ADAMTS13 levels were not available for all other cases making clear distinction between TTP and HUS difficult. We therefore analyzed results under the broader umbrella of TMA. In this context, we used a composite term TTP-HUS for clinical description.

3. Discussion

IFNs are a family of natural cytokines that interfere with viral replication, cell proliferation and immune regulation. Endogenous interferon production constitutes the initial nonspecific immune response against viral infections before specific host immune repertoire takes over. There are two major types of endogenous interferons: type 1 (IFNα—produced by leukocytes; IFNβ—produced by fibroblasts and epithelial cells) and type 2 (IFNγ—produced by activated T cells and NK cells). Viral infection activates pattern recognition receptors such as toll-like receptors (TLR) on macrophages and induces early IFN-1 activation. This further accelerates viral clearance by the upregulation of adaptive immune response [47]. Clinical applications of treatment with exogenous IFN include hematologic malignancies such as CML, lymphoma, PV; solid tumors such as renal cell carcinoma; and nonmalignant disorders such as MS and HCV. Besides CML and one case each of Sezary syndrome and hairy cell leukemia, IFN use has not been associated with TMA in any other myeloid or lymphoid malignancy [46, 48–52].

In order to understand pathologic process involved, it is important to outline the known and proposed mechanisms of action of IFN. Recombinant type I interferons (α and β) are pleiotropic cytokines that affect cellular function via immune regulatory mechanisms along with the regulation of cellular proliferation, apoptosis and angiogenesis. Dominant mechanisms are also disease specific. For example, in MS, T regulatory cell (Treg) dysregulation and decreased T helper (Th1) activity have been associated with clinical relapses [53]. Also, more recently, immunopathologic response from Th17 expansion and breakdown of blood brain barrier (BBB) have been implicated. Among other mechanisms, recombinant IFNβ is thought to restore Th1/Th2 balance, Treg function and regulation of T cell trafficking across BBB, thereby decreasing neuronal damage.

IFN action in myeloproliferative neoplasms (MPNs) is more complex, is incompletely understood and appears to utilize several pathways. While IFNα is not a Janus kinase 2 (JAK-2) inhibitor, it is able to eliminate the malignant JAK 2 mutant clone and achieve molecular remission in PV. There are a few widely accepted hypotheses for the mechanism of action of IFNα in MPN: enhanced cycling of quiescent leukemic stem cells (LSCs), restoration of dendritic cell function and promoting T cell activation by overcoming T cell energy [54–56].

Several possible pathophysiologic mechanisms have been described by which IFN may lead to TMA. In our review, cases with a clear diagnosis of TTP (with measured low levels of ADAMTS 13) also had ADAMTS 13 antibodies (ADAMTS 13 inhibitor). It appears that IFN-induced immune response plays a pivotal role in the production of cross-reacting anti-ADAMTS-13 antibodies with resultant microangiopathic hemolysis. While seemingly speculative, this observation has to be seen in the context of association of interferon therapy with the development of other autoimmune diseases. Prospective studies from patients treated with IFNα for hepatitis C showed that approximately 40% patients developed antithyroid antibodies with 15% developing clinical disease [57]. There are three different types of thyroid dysfunction associated with the IFN treatment: autoimmune (often subclinical) hypothyroidism, destructive thyroiditis and Graves hyperthyroidism. Females carry a higher risk to develop autoimmune thyroid disorders (AITDs) upon IFN treatment, with a relative risk of 4.4 (95% CI, 3.2–5.9) [58]. The pattern of thyroid disease observed resembles endogenous immunostimulation in the postpartum period. Development of multiple sclerosis has also been reported following the treatment of chronic phase CML with IFNα2b [59]. Taken together, these observations lend support to our inference that immune activation is fundamental for IFN-induced TTP.

The pathogenesis of TMA may also involve inhibition of vascular endothelial growth factor (VEGF) in renal podocytes [60]. Under physiologic conditions, VEGF stimulates signal transduction pathways and transcription through activation of its receptor VEGFR2. These events are essential for angiogenesis. The physiologic role of VEGF in kidneys is unclear but it has been associated with the pathophysiology of various renal diseases. Renal consequences of VEGF inhibition have been studied for VEGF antagonist bevacizumab. It has been proposed that local production of VEGF plays a critical protective role in microangiopathic processes. VEGF inhibitors such as bevacizumab disrupt this pathway and promote thrombotic microangiopathy [61]. IFN type 1 family also causes VEGF inhibition and hence may have a shared pathogenetic mechanism with VEGF antagonists. Vasoconstrictive and pro-coagulant effects of type I interferon have also been studied in pulmonary arterial hypertension. Experimental models have shown that IFNα increases pulmonary vascular resistance by the activation of thromboxane cascade [62].

There are various mechanisms proposed for IFN-induced HUS. Increased leukocyte adhesion to endothelial cells triggers endothelial damage and releases large multimers of von Willebrand factor causing endothelial swelling, platelet aggregation and intraluminal microthrombi formation causing tissue injury [63]. The development of antiphospholipid antibodies [64], antiendothelial cell antibodies and overexpression of class I antigens rendering cells vulnerable to cytotoxic response are some of the other described mechanisms [65].

Kavanagh et al. described potential immune-mediated and toxic mechanisms of IFN-induced TMA in MS patients [66]. They also reported a cumulative dose-toxicity relationship similar to our observation. In their analysis of data from a single institution involving eight patients, the duration of exposure was similar for IFNα and IFNβ, with TMA developing with long-term therapy at higher doses. In our analysis of a larger patient cohort, however, there is a statistically significant difference between the duration of exposure in MS (treated with IFNβ) versus CML and HCV (treated with IFNα). Although there is a complex interplay of a multitude of factors, our observations suggest that the underlying disease process is a key determinant accounting for the differences in the duration of exposure to IFN preceding onset of TMA. Additionally, however, the differences in IFN subtype (due to the differences in potencies of immunomodulatory and antiproliferative properties) is probably an additional, but secondary factor. In MS, among the accepted underlying mechanisms of IFN action is the ability to regain immunologic balance by restoring Treg cell function. On the other hand, in CML, IFN treatment creates a proinflammatory state for effective immune surveillance. This is supported by the observation of clonal T cell expansion in CML patients treated with IFNα. This difference between immune modulation and immune escalation could possibly account for the earlier development of TMA in CML. Similarly, in treatment of HCV, exogenous IFN binds to cell surface receptors and causes activation of IFN response genes (IRGs) via signal transduction through JAK–STAT pathway. This augments inflammatory response creating an antiviral state [67]. Immune dysfunction is commonly seen in lymphoproliferative disorders wherein the malignant cells originate from the immune system itself. It is therefore possible that impaired autoantibody production in this setting may be the reason for the lack of any observed cases of TMA in lymphoma. Limited clinical indications for IFN use may explain similar finding in PV.

Early diagnosis and prompt institution of treatment is of paramount importance in TMA. In contrast to drug-induced thrombocytopenia, IFN-induced TMA is insidious in onset with long incubation periods (average 40.2 months) and may masquerade as a more benign condition. It is therefore imperative that this association is recognized in clinical practice. Since ADAMTS13 results are not available in real time, a proposed quick guide to determine the likelihood of severely deficient ADAMTS13 activity is PLASMIC score (platelets, lysis, active cancer, stem cell or solid organ transplant, MCV, INR, creatinine): 0–4 score is associated with a low risk of severe ADAMTS13 deficiency, 5 score with intermediate risk and 6–7 scores with high risk [68].

Determining appropriate treatment for drug-associated TMA is challenging. Discontinuation of offending medication is the logical first step. Plasma exchange remains the standard treatment for acquired TTP. That said, since antibodies are present in only a small proportion of drug-associated TMA, the efficacy of plasma exchange in this setting is unclear [66]. A novel upcoming treatment option for patients with acquired TTP is Caplacizumab. This anti-von Willebrand factor (vWF) humanized immunoglobulin blocks vWF-mediated plasma aggregation and showed a 67% reduction in recurrence, 74% reduction in TTP-related death and a trend toward faster normalization of the three organ damage markers: lactate dehydrogenase (LDH), troponin and serum creatinine in the double-blind, placebo-controlled, phase 3 HERCULES trial [69]. These novel strategies may be a harbinger for new, more effective therapeutic options in TTP.

In the past few decades, most of the reported cases of IFN-induced TMA have been associated with CML, MS and chronic hepatitis C. Tyrosine kinase inhibitors are now the treatment standard for CML. Therefore, not surprisingly, there have been no reports of IFN-induced TMA in patients with CML in the last decade. In addition, with the development of more effective antiviral agents, interferon-free regimens for chronic hepatitis C are emerging. Taken together, with diminishing clinical applications of IFN, we may see an overall decrease in the reports of IFN-induced TMA hereon. The last few years, however, have also seen the emergence of immunooncology in cancer therapeutics. Immune checkpoint inhibitors including CTLA-4 antibodies and PD-1 ligands are now approved with expanding clinical applications. These agents potentiate immune response against tumors exponentially by blocking the inhibitory pathways utilized by tumors to escape host immune surveillance mechanisms. Augmentation of host immunity, however, results in breaking self-tolerance and induction of immune-related side effects (ir-AE). Most common side effects are colitis and pneumonitis requiring immune suppression for resolution. Cortazar et al. described a 58-year-old male with melanoma who developed TMA that correlated with treatment with Ipilimumab (CTLA-4 antibody) [70]. This is an interesting observation in the context of our analysis, especially of the mechanisms involved in IFN-induced TMA. It is yet to be ascertained, as we gain more experience with these agents whether this will be an isolated or consistent observation. Nevertheless, it would be prudent to consider the likelihood of these adverse effects in the future.

4. Conclusion

Historically, exogenous IFN (α and β) has been the primary therapy for a variety of diseases such as chronic HCV, chronic phase CML, MS, lymphoma and PV. IFN can trigger autoimmune diseases such as autoimmune thyroiditis. IFN-mediated immune upregulation with the production of cross-reacting antibodies to ADAMTS 13 and complement activation from endothelial injury are the probable pathways for IFN-induced TMA. From our observation, barring differences in time of onset and cumulative dose exposure, the presentation, clinical course and response to treatment appear to be similar among different IFN subtypes and across all indications of use. Treatment regimens utilizing plasma exchange, steroids and rituximab result in durable responses. While interferon may have a myelosuppressive effect causing gradual onset thrombocytopenia, thrombotic microangiopathy, a possible fatal complication should be considered in the differential diagnosis. Once recognized, early institution of appropriate treatment results in favorable outcome. Our analysis also indicates that in patients who had positive ADAMTS13 inhibitors, plasma exchange was a very effective therapy with complete response. Finally, while interferons may have diminishing clinical applications, interferon-induced thrombotic microangiopathy has provided us with valuable lessons pertaining to collateral consequences of immune upregulation. This has resulted in a paradigm shift in our understanding of immunobiology and will have far reaching applications in immunomodulating therapeutics.

Acknowledgements

Vladimir Gotlieb, MD, Boris Avezbakiyev, MD, Hesham Taha, MD, Brookdale University Hospital Medical Center, Brooklyn, NY, USA.

Conflict of interest

None.

Author details

Ajay Kundra[1], Mirela Andrei[2] and Jen Chin Wang[3*]

*Address all correspondence to: jcwang0005@gmail.com

1 Providence Regional Medical Center, Everett, WA, USA

2 St Mary's Regional Medical Center, Lewiston, ME, USA

3 Division of Hematology/Oncology, Brookdale University Hospital Medical Center, Brooklyn, NY, USA

References

[1] Scully M. Thrombocytopenia in hospitalized patients: approach to the patient with thrombotic microangiopathy. In: American Society of Hematology 59th Annual Meeting & Exposition. Atlanta, GA: American Society of Hematology Education Program; 2017 Dec 8;**2017**(1):651-659. DOI: 10.1182/asheducation-2017.1.651

[2] Kundra A, Wang JC. Interferon induced thrombotic microangiopathy (TMA): Analysis and concise review. Critical Reviews in Oncology/Hematology. 2017;**112**:103-112

[3] Poddar N, Wang JC. Thrombotic thrombocytopenic purpura in a patient with interferon treated hepatitis C successfully treated with rituximab. Hematology Reports. 2013;**5**(1):5-7

[4] Schlaifer D, Dumazer P, Spenatto N, Mignon-Conte M, Brousset P, Lumbroso C, Cooper M, Muller C, Huguet F, Attal M, et al. Hemolytic-uremic syndrome in a patient with chronic myelogenous leukemia treated with interferon alpha. American Journal of Hematology. 1994 Nov;**47**(3):254-255

[5] Harvey M, Rosenfeld D, Davies D, Hall BM. Recombinant interferon alpha and hemolytic uremic syndrome: cause or coincidence? American Journal of Hematology. 1994 Jun;**46**(2):152-153

[6] Jadoul M, Piessevaux H, Ferrant A, Cosyns JP, van Ypersele de Strihou C. Renal thrombotic microangiopathy in patients with chronic myelogenous leukaemia treated with interferon-alpha 2b. Nephrology, Dialysis, Transplantation. 1995;**10**(1):111-113

[7] Lipton JH, Minden M. CML may not be part of HUS. American Journal of Hematology. May 1995;**49**(1):100-101

[8] Honda K, Ando A, Endo M, Shimizu K, Higashihara M, Nitta K, Nihei H. Thrombotic microangiopathy associated with alpha-interferon therapy for chronic myelocytic leukemia. American Journal of Kidney Diseases. Jul 1997;**30**(1):123-130

[9] Rachmani R, Avigdor A, Youkla M, Raanani P, Zilber M, Ravid M, Ben-Bassat I. Thrombotic thrombocytopenic purpura complicating chronic myelogenous leukemia treated with interferon-alpha. A report of two successfully treated patients. Acta Haematologica. 1998;**100**(4):204-206

[10] Vacher-Coponat H, Opris A, Daniel L, Harle J-R, Veit V, Olmer M. Thrombotic microangiopathy in a patient with chronic myelocytic leukaemia treated with α-interferon. Nephrology Dialysis Transplantation. 1999;**14**:2469-2471

[11] Ravandi-Kashani F, Cortes J, Talpaz M, Kantarijan H. Thrombotic microangiopathy associated with interferon therapy for patients with chronic myelogenous leukemia. Cancer. 1999;**85**:2583-2588

[12] Lacotte L, Thierry A, Delwail V, Dreyfus B, Guilhot F. Thrombotic thrombocytopenic purpura during interferon alpha treatment for chronic myelogenous leukemia. Acta Haematologica. 1999;**102**:160-162

[13] Magee CC, Abraham K, Farrell J, Dorman T, Walshe JJ. Renal thrombotic microangiopathy associated with interferon-alpha treatment of chronic myeloid leukemia. American Journal of Kidney Diseases. Jul 2000;**36**(1):E5

[14] Denizon N, Beraud JJ, Mourad G, Blanc P, Bureau JP, Navarro M, Lavabre-Bertrand T. Hemolitic uremic syndrome with hypertransaminasemia following treatment by interferon

for chronic myeloid leukemia. Gastroentérologie Clinique et Biologique. Nov 2001;**25**(11): 1039-1040

[15] Badid C, McGregor B, Marie Faivre J, Guerard A, Juillard L, Fouque D, Laville M. Renal thrombotic microangiopathy induced by interferon-α. Nephrology Dialysis Transplantation. 2001;**16**:846-848

[16] Zuber J, Martinez F, Droz D, Oksenhendler E, Legendre C. Alpha-interferon-associated thrombotic microangiopathy: A clinicopathologic study of 8 patients and review of literature. Medicine. July 2002;**81**(4):321-331

[17] Ohashi N, Yonemura K, Sugiura T, Isozaki T, Togawa A, Fujigaki Y, Yamamoto T, Hishida A. Withdrawal of interferon-alpha results in prompt resolution of thrombocytopenia and hemolysis but not renal failure in hemolytic uremic syndrome caused by interferon-alpha. American Journal of Kidney Diseases. Mar 2003;**41**(3):E10

[18] Galesic K, Bozic B, Racic I, Scukanec-Spoljar M. Thrombotic microangiopathy associated with alpha-interferon therapy for chronic myeloid leukaemia. Nephrology (Carlton, Vic.). Feb 2006;**11**(1):49-52

[19] Herrera WG, Balizet LB, Harberts SW, Brown ST. Occurrence of a TTP-like syndrome in two women receiving beta interferon therapy for relapsing multiple sclerosis. Neurology. Apr 1999;**52**(6 supplement 2):A135

[20] Serrano A, Xicoy B, Grifols JR, Ribera JM. Thrombotic thrombocytopenic purpura during treatment with interpheron. Medicina clínica (Barc). 2007;**128**(7):276-277 (Spanish)

[21] Li Cavoli G, Bono L, Tortorici C, Giammarresi C, Rotolo U. Renal thrombotic microangiopathy induced by β-interferon. NDT Plus. 2011;**4**(1):80-80

[22] Broughton A, Cosyns J-P, Jadoul M. Thrombotic microangiopathy induced by long-term interferon-β therapy for multiple sclerosis: a case report. Clinical Nephrology. Nov 2011;**76**(5):396-400

[23] Bensa C, Sohier E, Pillebout L, Galicier L, Gout O. A case of thrombotic microangiopathy associated with subcutaneous beta-1a-interferon therapy. Multiple Sclerosis. 2011;**17**:S227

[24] Olea T, Díaz-Mancebo R, Picazo M-L, Jorge M-A, Robles A, Selgas R. Thrombotic microangiopathy associated with use of interferon-beta. International Journal of Nephrology and Renovascular Disease. 2012;**5**:97-100

[25] Modrego PJ, Gazulla J. Arterial hypertension induced by interferon beta 1b in a patient with multiple sclerosis. Multiple Sclerosis Journal. 2012;**18**(11):1655-1656

[26] Nerrant E, Charif M, Ramay AS, Perrochia H, Patrier L, de Champfleur NM, Renard D, Labauge P. Hemolytic uremic syndrome: An unusual complication of interferon-β treatment in a MS patient. Journal of Neurology. Jul 2013;**260**(7):1915-1916. DOI: 10.1007/s00415-013-6961-8 [Epub May 25, 2013]

[27] Mahe J, Meurette A, Moreau A, Vercel C, Jolliet P. Renal thrombotic microangiopathy caused by interferon beta-1a treatment for multiple sclerosis. Drug Design, Development and Therapy. Aug 7, 2013;**7**:723-728

[28] Larochelle C, Grand'maison F, Bernier GP, Latour M, Cailhier JF, Prat A. Thrombotic thrombocytopenic purpura- hemolytic uremic syndrome in relapsing-remitting multiple sclerosis patients on high dose interferon β. Multiple Sclerosis. 2014;(13):1783-1787

[29] Orvain C, Augusto J-F, Besson V, Marc G, Coppo P, Subra J-F, Sayegh J. Thrombotic microangiopathy due to acquired ADAMTS13 deficiency in a patient receiving interferon-beta treatment for multiple sclerosis. International Urology and Nephrology. 2014;**46**:239-242

[30] Vosoughi R, Marriott J. Thrombotic microangiopathy in Interferon Beta treated multiple sclerosis patients: review of literature and report of two new cases. Multiple Sclerosis and Related Disorders. May 2014;**3**:321-325

[31] Hunt D, Kavanagh D, Drummond L, Overell J, Evans S, Jackson A, Chandran S. Thrombotic microangiopathy associated with interferon beta. New England Journal of Medicine. Mar 27, 2014;**370**:1270-1271

[32] Kobayashi H, Utsunomiya Y, Miyazaki Y, Tokutome G, Kawamura T, Hashimoto T, Sakai T, Takahashi S, Tojyo A, Asano S. Case of chronic myelogenous leukemia with hemolytic-uremic-syndrome like kidney during long-term interferon-alpha therapy. Nihon Naika Gakkai Zasshi. Jul 10, 1997;**86**(7):1259-1261

[33] Ubara Y, Hara S, Takedatu H, Katori H, Yamada K, Yoshihara K, Matsushita Y, Yokoyama K, Takemoto F, Yamada A, Takagawa R, Endo Y, Hara M, Koida I, Kumada H. Hemolytic uremic syndrome associated with beta-interferon therapy for chronic hepatitis C. Nephron. Sep 1998;**80**(1):107-108

[34] Iyoda K, Kato M, Nakagawa T, Kakiuchi Y, Sugiyasu Y, Fujii E, et al. Thrombotic thrombocytopenic purpura developed suddenly during interferon treatment for chronic hepatitis C. Journal of Gastroenterology. 1998;**33**(4):588-592

[35] Creput C, Auffret N, Samuel D, Jian R, Hill G, Nochy D. Cutaneous thrombotic microangiopathy during treatment with alpha-interferon for chronic hepatitis C. Journal of Hepatology. Dec 2002;**37**(6):871-872

[36] Kitano K, Gibo Y, Kamijo A, Furuta K, Oguchi S, Joshita S, Takahashi Y, Ishida F, Matsumoto M, Uemura M, Fujimura Y. Thrombotic thrombocytopenic purpura associated with pegylated-interferon alpha-2a by an ADAMTS13 inhibitor in a patient with chronic hepatitis C. Haematologica. 2006;**91**(8 Suppl):ECR34

[37] Deutsch M, Manesis EK, Hadziyannis E, Vassilopoulos D, Archimandritis AJ. Thrombotic thrombocytopenic purpura with fatal outcome in a patient with chronic hepatitis C treated with pegylated interferon-a/2b. Scandinavian Journal of Gastroenterology. 2007;**42**(3):408-409

[38] Sallée M, Crétel E, Jean R, Chiche L, Bourlière M, Poullin P, et al. Thrombotic thrombocytopenic purpura complicating interferon therapy in chronic C hepatitis. Gastroentérologie Clinique et Biologique. 2008;**32**(2):145-146

[39] Hepburn IS, Schade R. Thrombotic thrombocytopenic purpura (TTP) associated with interferon therapy of hepatitis C. Grand Rounds. 2010;**10**:1-7

[40] Lambot F, Hanson B, Sztern B. Thrombotic thrombocytopenic purpura mediated by an ADAMTS13-inhibitor related to a treatment with peglyated-interferon alpha-2a and ribavarine in a patient with chronic hepatitis C. La Presse Médicale. 2010;**39**(11):1207-1210

[41] Iskander D, Wickremasinghe M, Bain BJ. Thrombotic microangiopathy complicating pegylated interferon treatment of hepatitis C infection. American Journal of Hematology. Oct 2011;**86**(10):859

[42] Michaux C, Randrianasolo D, Vandenhende MA, Hessamfar M, Morlat P, Bonnet F. Thrombotic thrombocytopenic purpura associated with interferon therapy in a HIV and HCV co-infected woman. Revue de Médecine Interne. 2013;**34**(12):773-775

[43] Boctor FN, Chiosea I, Bradley T. Thrombotic thrombocytopenic purpura with unusual 33 recurrences: A case report. Annals of Clinical and Laboratory Science. 2013;**43**(1):91-93

[44] Evans R, Pavan M, Suri D, Harber M. Thrombotic microangiopathy (TMA) in a patient treated with antiviral therapy for hepatitis C. BML Case Reports. Apr 2014;**4**:2014

[45] Stratta P, Canavese C, Dogliani M, Thea A, Degani G, Mairone L, Vercellone A. Hemolytic-uremic syndrome during recombinant alpha-interferon treatment for hairy cell leukemia. Renal Failure. 1993;**15**(4):559-561

[46] Politou M, Tsaftarides P, Vassiliades J, Siakantaris M, Michail S, Nakopoulou L, Pangalis G, Vaiopoulos G. Thrombotic microangiopathy in a patient with Sezary syndrome treated with interferon-α. Nephrology Dialysis Transplantation. March 2004;**19**(3):733-735

[47] Rosen HR. Chronic hepatitis C infection. The New England Journal of Medicine. 2011;**364**:2429-2438

[48] Foon KA, Roth MS, Bunn Jr PA. Interferon therapy of non-Hodgkin's lymphoma. Cancer. 1987;**59**(Suppl):601-604

[49] Avilés A. The role of interferon as maintenance therapy in malignant lymphoma. Medical Oncology. 1997;**14**:153-157

[50] Gaynor ER, Fisher RI. Clinical trials of alpha-interferon in the treatment of non-Hodgkin's lymphoma. Seminars in Oncology. 1991;**18**(Suppl 7):12-17

[51] Silver RT. Interferon-2b: A new treatment for Polycythemia Vera. Annals of Internal Medicine. 1993;**119**(11):1091-1092

[52] Tefferi A, Elliott MA. Interferon-alpha therapy in polycythemia vera and essential thrombocythemia. Seminars in Thrombosis and Hemostasis. 1997;**23**:463-472

[53] Kieseier BC. The mechanism of action of interferon-β in relapsing multiple sclerosis. CNS Drugs. June 2011;**25**(6):491-502

[54] Burchert A, Saussele S, Eigendorff E, Müller MC, Sohlbach K, Inselmann S, Schütz C, Metzelder SK, Ziermann J, Kostrewa P, Hoffmann J, Hehlmann R, Neubauer A. Hochhaus A Interferon alpha 2 maintenance therapy may enable high rates of treatment discontinuation in chronic myeloid leukemia. Leukemia. Jun 2015;**29**(6):1331-1335

[55] Kiladjian JJ, Giraudier S, Cassinat B. Interferon-alpha for the therapy of myeloproliferative neoplasms: targeting the malignant clone. Leukemia. 2016;**30**:776-781

[56] Brown S, Hutchinson CV, Aspinall-O'Dea M, Whetton AD, Johnson SM, Rees-Unwin K, Burthem J. Monocyte-derived dendritic cells from chronic myeloid leukaemia have abnormal maturation and cytoskeletal function that is associated with defective localisation and signalling by normal ABL1 protein. European Journal of Haematology. Aug 2014;**93**(2):96-102

[57] Mandac JC, Chaudhry S, Sherman KE, Tomer Y. The clinical and physiological spectrum of interferon-alpha induced thyroiditis. Toward a new classification. Hepatology. 2006;**43**(4):661-672

[58] Fattovich G, Giustina G, Favarato S, Ruol A. Investigators of the Italian Association for the Study of the Liver. A survey of adverse events in 11,241 patients with chronic viral hepatitis treated with alfa interferon. Journal of Hepatology. 1996;**24**:38-47

[59] Kataoka I, Shinagawa K, Shiro Y, Okamoto S, Watanabe R, Mori T, Ito D, Harada M. Multiple sclerosis associated with interferon-alpha therapy for chronic myelogenous leukemia. American Journal of Hematology. 2002;**70**(2):149-153

[60] George JN, Terrell DR, Vesely SK, Kremer Hovinga JA, Lämmle B. Thrombotic microangiopathic syndromes associated with drugs, HIV infection, hematopoietic stem cell transplantation and cancer. Presse Médicale. Mar 2012;**41**(3 Pt 2):e177-e188

[61] Eremina V, Jefferson A, Kowalewska J, Hochster H, Haas M, Weisstuch J, Richardson C, Kopp JB, Kabir MG, Backx P, Gerber HP, Ferrara N, Barisoni L, Alpers CE, Quaggin S. VEGF inhibition and renal thrombotic microangiopathy. The New England Journal of Medicine. 2008;**358**:1129-1136

[62] Rot U, Ledinek AH. Interferons beta have vasoconstrictive and procoagulant effects: a woman who developed livedo reticularis and Raynaud phenomenon in association with interferon beta treatment for multiple sclerosis. Clinical Neurology and Neurosurgery. 2013 Dec;**115**(Suppl 1):S79-S81

[63] Ruggenenti P, Noris M, Remuzzi G. Thrombotic microangiopathy, hemolytic hemolytic syndrome, and thrombotic thrombocytopenic purpura. Kidney International. 2001;831-846

[64] Piette JC, Papo T. Potential role for antiphospholipid antibodies in renal thrombotic microangiopathy induced by interferon-alpha. Nephrololgy Dialysis Transplantation. 1995;**10**(9):1781

[65] Leung DY, Moake JL, Havens PL, Kim M, Pober JS. Lytic anti-endothelial cell antibodies in haemolytic-uraemic syndrome. Lancet. 1988;**2**(8604):183-186

[66] Kavanagh D, McGlasson S, Jury A, Williams J, Scolding N, Bellamy C, Gunther C, Ritchie D, Gale DP, Kanwar YS, Challis R, Buist H, Overell J, Weller B, Flossmann O, Blunden M, Meyer EP, Krucker T, Evans SJ, Campbell IL, Jackson AP, Chandran S, Hunt DP. Type I interferon causes thrombotic microangiopathy by a dose-dependent toxic effect on the microvasculature. Blood. Dec 15, 2016;**128**(24):2824-2833

[67] Feld J, Hoofnagle J. Mechanism of action of interferon and ribavirin in treatment of hepatitis C. Nature. Aug 2005;**436**:967-972

[68] Bendapudi PK, Hurwitz S, Fry A, Marques MB, Waldo SW, Li A, Sun L, Upadhyay V, Hamdan A, Brunner AM, Gansner JM, Viswanathan S, Kaufman RM, Uhl L, Stowell CP, Dzik WH, Makar RS. Derivation and external validation of the PLASMIC score for rapid assessment of adults with thrombotic microangiopathies: A cohort study. Lancet Haematology. 2017;**4**(4):e157-e164

[69] Scully M, Cataland SR, Peyvandi F, et al. Results of the randomized, double-blind, placebo-controlled, phase 3 HERCULES study of capecitabine of caplacizumab in patients with aquired thrombotic thrombocytopenic purpura. Oral presentation at: American Society of Hematology 59th Annual Meeting & Exposition; 2017 December 9-12; Atlanta, GA

[70] Cortazar FB, Marrone KA, Troxell ML, Ralto KM, Hoenig MP, Brahmer JR, Le DT, Lipson EJ, Glezerman IG, Wolchok J, Cornell LD, Feldman P, Stokes MB, Zapata SA, Hodi FS, Ott PA, Yamashita M, Leaf DE. Clinicopathological features of acute kidney injury associated with immune checkpoint inhibitors. Kidney International. 2016 Sep;**90**(3):638-47. DOI: 10.1016/j.kint.2016.04.008. Epub 2016 Jun 7

Chapter 6

Thrombocytopenia in Liver Transplant

Gabriela Droc

Additional information is available at the end of the chapter

http://dx.doi.org/10.5772/intechopen.72510

Abstract

Thrombocytopenia is a common complication of both chronic liver disease and liver transplantation (LT). The mechanism of thrombocytopenia is multifactorial implicating not only sequestration in the spleen, or in the graft, reduction in the mean platelet survival but also decreased platelet production due to low synthesis of thrombopoietin (TPO) or direct toxicity to the bone marrow. Platelets play a dualistic role in liver transplant, both beneficial and detrimental. The beneficial role of platelets is due to platelet-derived serotonin that is involved in liver regeneration. During surgery for liver transplant, in addition to the preoperative causes for thrombocytopenia, we have other mechanisms that will contribute to further deterioration of the platelets count and function: hemodilution, immunological reactions, and sequestration in the newly transplanted graft. This might result in a life-threatening level of thrombocytes. The concern is when we should treat thrombocytopenia because despite life-saving benefits, transfusion has also been related to complications and platelet transfusion has been identified as an independent risk factor for postoperative complications. Risks related to platelet concentrate administration are allergic reactions, alloimmunization, bacterial sepsis, and transfusion-related acute lung injury (TRALI). Administration of platelets is not indicated if there is no bleeding or immediate bleeding risk. New emerging therapies like thrombopoietin-receptor agonist will furthermore limit the administration of blood products.

Keywords: thrombocytopenia, liver transplant, thrombopoietin, splenectomy, cirrhosis

1. Introduction

Thrombocytopenia is a common complication of both chronic liver disease and liver transplantation (LT) contributing to the complex hemostasis disturbances of those patients. Liver disease induces a complicated imbalance between pro- and antihemostatic elements, thrombocytopenia just being one of them. The mechanism of thrombocytopenia is multifactorial implicating not only sequestration in the spleen, reduction in the mean platelet survival but also decreased platelet production due to low synthesis of thrombopoietin (TPO) [1].

In chronic liver disease, a low platelet count is a marker of severity and is associated with poorer prognosis [2].

Liver transplantation (LT), the main treatment of end-stage liver disease, can also induce decrease of thrombocytes starting intraoperative with the reperfusion syndrome and going on after the procedure due to several mechanisms among which sequestration in the graft plays an important role [1]. Platelets have a dualistic role in LT, both beneficial and detrimental [3].

Thrombocytopenia is defined by platelet count <150,000/mm^3; it is mild if platelets are between 75,000 and 150,000/mm^3, moderate for values between 50,000 and 75,000/mm^3, and severe if the count is <50,000/mm^3. Definitions may vary and the limits of platelet count might be different in different studies [4].

The incidence of decreased platelets in chronic liver disease is as high as 76% but moderate in only 13% and severe in 1% of cirrhotic patients [5]. The degree of thrombocytopenia is dependent on the stage of cirrhosis. However, spontaneous bleeding does not occur unless the values reaches 10,000–20,000/mm^3. There is a difference if an invasive procedure such as liver biopsy, variceal ligation, paracentesis, or major surgery is intended; platelet threshold levels are higher and differ depending on the invasiveness of the maneuver. However, bleeding is not the only concern with thrombocytopenia as platelets have other roles in inflammation, angiogenesis, antimicrobial defense and, of specific importance, in ischemia/reperfusion injury and a beneficial role in liver regeneration [6].

2. Causes/mechanisms for thrombocytopenia in liver transplant

2.1. Thrombocytopenia and platelet dysfunction in liver disease

Platelet count, as well as their function, is altered in patients with cirrhosis in the waiting list for transplantation. The pathogenesis of this phenomenon is not well understood. There are several mechanisms implicated in this process: on one hand, depletion of platelets due to destruction and on the other, an altered production. The main cause seems to be platelet sequestration in the enlarged, congestive spleen due to portal hypertension.

Apart from **hypersplenism,** other causes are reduced production of platelets, low TPO levels, existence of antiplatelet antibodies, alcohol toxicity, folate deficiency, chronic low-grade disseminated intravascular coagulation, and direct viral suppression of platelet production as provided in **Table 1** [7, 8].

There is a strong correlation between spleen volume and thrombocytopenia, thus measures that aim to diminish hypersplenism will probably have a good impact on platelet count. Splenectomy prior to transplantation has been proposed as a therapeutic option to increase platelet count but this approach remains controversial because splenic pooling is not so significant as it was first described and the removal of the spleen does not always lead to

Mechanisms	
Altered production	Low TPO levels Bone marrow suppression (HCV, alcohol) Medication
Sequestration	Congestive spleen due to portal hypertension
Enhanced destruction/loss	Platelet antibodies Chronic low-grade disseminated intravascular coagulation Bleeding

Table 1. Causes for thrombocytopenia in chronic liver disease.

substantial and persistent increase in thrombocytes. On the other hand, elimination of the spleen increases the risk of septic complications and portal thrombosis [4].

Shunt procedures done either surgically or percutaneously [transjugular intrahepatic portosystemic shunt (TIPS)] are intended at decreasing portal hypertension and hypersplenism might also have a beneficial effect on platelet count. Massoud, following 92 patients that had a TIPS placement, reported a significant increase in platelet number after the procedure, this increase being more important in patients with more severe thrombocytopenia. But TIPS would not have any effect on TPO, this being a possible reason why in some cases there was no effect on platelet number [7].

Cirrhotic patients waiting for transplantation are sometimes in need for invasive procedures like liver biopsies, endoscopic variceal ligation, paracentesis, and transjugular intrahepatic portosystemic shunt. There is no absolute threshold of platelet count for performing any of those procedures but if platelets are <75,000/mm^3, the risk of bleeding seems to be higher [4].

Thrombocytopenia was also a concern in patients with hepatitis C virus (HCV), who needed antiviral therapy with interferon and had to reduce doses or even stop treatment. Nowadays with the new antiviral therapies, this should not be a problem anymore.

TPO is a thrombopoietic hormone produced in the liver by both parenchymal cells and sinusoidal endothelial cells at a constant rate. The blood level of TPO is dependent on the uptake by platelets and megakaryocytes, where it is destroyed so if platelet count decreases, less TPO will be uptake and destroyed and its level will rise. Production of TPO is dependent on liver cell integrity; if that is impaired, production will decrease as in cirrhosis. This explains why with a reduction in platelet number TPO level in liver disease would not be elevated, as production is lower. TPO level is inappropriate to platelet level and as a consequence the bone marrow stimulation to produce thrombocytes would not be adequate [2, 4].

Antiplatelet antibodies contribute to the premature destruction of the thrombocytes. It was shown among patients with liver disease that up to 64% irrespective of the etiology have platelet-associated anti-glycoprotein (anti-GP) antibodies that are directed against the GP IIb-IX complex. The serum of those patients also has higher levels of platelet-associated immunoglobulin G also implicated in the immune-mediated destruction of platelets [2].

Decreased platelet production by the bone marrow is also one of the mechanisms implicated in thrombocytopenia of chronic liver disease. HCV directly inhibits the growth and differentiation of bone marrow stem cells and alcohol leads to ineffective megakaryopoiesis. Production of platelets is also inhibited by some of the medication those patients might need, for example, interferon [2].

Bleeding is not as frequent in cirrhotic patients as one can imagine and that can be explained by some compensatory mechanisms. Part of the complex problem of platelet function in cirrhosis is the demonstrated capacity of platelets to sustain thrombin generation at an equal level with control if adjusted to normal levels. This concludes that their function might not be as altered as primary thought [9]. And there are compensatory mechanisms to bleeding disorders of the cirrhotic patient, one of them being the elevated level of von Willebrand factor reaching 10-fold the plasma level of control and supporting platelet adhesion better than in healthy volunteers [3, 10].

2.2. Intraoperative challenges

Liver transplantation is a huge challenge with any anesthesiologist for two main problems such as hemodynamic changes during surgery and coagulation status of the patient. Surgery consists of three phases: removal of the cirrhotic liver during which, due to portal hypertension, there is a high bleeding risk aggravated by the patients' coagulopathy; the anhepatic phase with hemodynamic disturbances; and the neohepatic phase that starts with the reperfusion of the graft inducing hypotension, cardiac rhythm disturbances, and impacts on coagulation.

During surgery, in addition to the preoperative causes for thrombocytopenia, we have other mechanisms that will contribute to further deterioration of the platelets count and function such as bleeding, hemodilution, immunological reactions, and sequestration in the newly transplanted graft [3].

Several authors present the hypothesis that removal of the spleen during LT procedure will ameliorate platelet count. Ohira et al. [11] reported an analysis of the relationship between preoperative spleen volume and thrombocytopenia and suggested that splenectomy might be considered simultaneously with LT in chronic hepatitis C virus (HCV) patients with a preoperative platelet count of <60,000/mm^3. The intent is to facilitate an interferon therapy immediately after LT. Almost all recipients will have a reinfection of the graft with HCV; they need antiviral therapy during the postoperative period but this might be impossible to apply due to thrombocytopenia. However, there are risks related to splenectomy; patients are prone to develop portal vein thrombosis and have a higher risk for infection and sepsis.

Morimoto et al. [12] analyzed their results for 36 patients undergoing LT and reported similar conclusions. Their criteria for performing splenectomy were a platelet count <50,000/mm^3 and a spleen volume reported to the body surface area of >400 ml/m^2 and so it was done in six patients, all of them completing their interferon therapy after LT. They registered only one systemic infection possibly related to splenectomy.

In the publication by Chu et al. addressing 40 patients selected for splenectomy during LT because they had HCV infection associated with hypersplenism or they were expected to develop small-for-size syndrome or they had huge spleens that affected surgical maneuvers during transplant. In this selected group of patients, the authors indicated that simultaneous splenectomy did not increase the rate of perioperative complications or risk of mortality [13].

All the authors do not have the same opinion. In a recently published study recording 169 patients who underwent living-related LT with splenectomy [14], the authors found that concomitant splenectomy with LT surgery did not increase platelet count in the early postoperative period but they had more reinterventions due to hemorrhage, the operative time was longer, intraoperative blood loss was higher, and the incidence of lethal infectious disease was higher when compared to patients not having splenectomy during living donor LT.

Reperfusion of the graft is one of the most delicate moments during transplant surgery resulting not only in hemodynamic changes but also in alterations of the circulating platelets. Decreased aggregation of thrombocytes has been observed after reperfusion of the liver with a peak value within 1 hour and postoperative reduction in platelet surface markers glycoprotein (GP) IIb/IIa and P selectin [15]. Secondary to ischemia/reperfusion, platelets will suffer in number and function. They undergo a decrease by 30–55% due to entrapment in the graft. Platelets will adhere to the sinusoidal endothelium that has been activated during the cold and warm ischemia and will induce direct injury to the liver cell [3].

There is also a rare condition that might lead to severe thrombocytopenia after transplantation such as de novo development of idiopathic thrombocytopenic purpura [3].

2.3. Postoperative outcome

After transplantation, thrombocytopenia occurs during the first days and is a common disorder. The lowest values are observed on days 3–5 and if no complication happens, the resolution of the process will start after the first week. The main mechanism implicated in this thrombocytopenia is the sequestration of the platelets in the graft (**Table 2**). However, the lowest the platelets count in this period, the most severe and complicated the course of the posttransplant period [16].

Mechanisms	
Altered production	Bone marrow suppression (medication)
Sequestration	Liver graft
Enhanced destruction/loss	Bleeding
	Infectious complications
	Platelet antibodies
	Heparin-induced

Table 2. Causes for thrombocytopenia post liver transplant.

Lesurtel et al. proposed a new criterion in evaluating the extent and impact of thrombocytopenia they called the 60-5 criterion. In their study, they demonstrated a strong correlation between a platelet count of <60,000/mm^3 on postoperative day 5 and the incidence of severe complications and a twofold increase in mortality at 90 days [17].

A rare cause of low platelet count in this stage is heparin-induced thrombocytopenia, heparin therapy being the standard of care in many centers post LT. Bachmann et al. in a single center study looking at 205 LT found in 1.95% of patients, a suspicious clinical platelet course with elevated antibody levels [18].

Chang et al. looked at the role platelets have in antimicrobial host defense. They analyzed 50 LT recipients and looked at the impact of thrombocytopenia as a related variable to infectious complications in the posttransplant period. They found a significant correlation between low platelet count (<30,000/mm^3) and infections in the first month following transplantation. The correlation was very strong for fungal and bacterial infections but not for viral ones. Infection can determine thrombocytopenia but the authors stated that the lowest platelet count preceded the infection with a median time of 7 days [19].

Generally, platelet transfusion is not needed during the postoperative period and one can wait for the spontaneous resolution. Resolution starts after the first week due to increasing levels of thrombopoietin. It will reach normal values on time due to the regression of splenomegaly once portal hypertension has been resolved [20].

After liver transplantation, the blood level of TPO increases but it will take several days for the rise of platelet number to happen [21].

The **beneficial role** of platelets is due to platelet-derived serotonin that is involved in liver regeneration. This phenomenon is of great importance in living-related LT, small-for-size syndrome, and also plays a role in hepatic repair after ischemia/reperfusion injury. Serotonin accumulates in thrombocytes and is released in areas of tissue injury stimulating mitogenesis [3]. All the mechanisms promoting liver regeneration and involving platelets are not yet very well understood but they certainly play an important role through the release of various mediators like serotonin, hepatocyte growth factor, insulin growth factor, and vascular endothelial growth factor. The last one supports liver regeneration by stimulating neoangiogenesis [22].

3. Treating thrombocytopenia

Blood loss is a major concern during liver transplantation due to the precarious hemostatic condition of these patients combined to a surgical procedure at high risk for bleeding. Since the beginnings of LT, surgical techniques and anesthetic patient management have improved and the blood loss and transfusion needs have decreased. Despite life-saving benefits, transfusion has also related complications and platelet transfusion has been identified as an independent risk factor for postoperative complications. Risks related to platelet concentrate administration are allergic reactions, alloimmunization, bacterial sepsis, and transfusion-related acute lung injury (TRALI), and nowadays to a lesser extent viral transmission [23]. Therapeutic rather than prophylactic administration of platelets concentrate is recommended with a possible threshold of 50,000/mm^3 during surgery associated with diffuse bleeding [24].

In a study analyzing possible complications related to platelet administration during LT, Pereboom [25] has shown that patients who received platelet concentrates had lower patient and graft survival than patients who had only blood loss or low level of thrombocytes but were not transfused with platelets. Their main complication was related to platelet transfusion and at the same time the specific cause of death was TRALI. TRALI is more frequently associated with plasma-rich blood products such as platelet concentrates and fresh frozen plasma and this might be related to the growth of inflammatory mediators in the stored platelets. It has been shown that cytokine levels are 1000-fold greater in stored platelets when compared to healthy volunteers and this might be related to the fact that platelets need to be kept at room temperature that also makes them prone to bacterial contamination. One could argue that transfusion needs are related to sicker patients but the author has shown that survival rates for those patients with severe blood loss and a low platelet count are similar to reference population if they were not transfused with platelet concentrates [25].

Despite the general consensus that platelet transfusions are related to worse outcome, there is a type of LT, the living-related LT where recipients might benefit from exogenous thrombocytes. Kim et al. on a series of 227 living-related LT conducted a study to define the effects of platelet transfusion on the liver regeneration and reached the conclusion that it has a beneficial effect [26].

The use of blood products and fibrinogen concentrate following a thrombelastometry-guided protocol (TEG/ROTEM) has led to a decrease in overall transfusion requirements, platelet concentrates as well, by offering a picture of the complete coagulation process with information on the dynamics of clot formation [27, 28].

Eltrombopag is an oral thrombopoietin-receptor agonist still looking for its place in the treatment of thrombocytopenia in chronic liver disease. It has got an indication for patients with chronic HCV infection for the initiation or maintenance of interferon therapy. Afdhal et al. published in the name of the ELEVATE study group a paper showing that eltrombopag reduced the need for platelet transfusion in liver disease patients undergoing invasive procedures [29].

4. Conclusion

In conclusion, thrombocytopenia is a common figure of chronic liver disease and liver transplant with multifactorial etiologies. Platelet count exclusively is not a good marker to anticipate risk for bleeding in cirrhotic patients because compensatory mechanisms increasing production of von Willebrand factor will interfere. Splenectomy is not indicated anymore as a therapeutic measure for regulating thrombocytopenia in the pretransplant period. It still may have some indications if done concomitantly with the transplant procedure especially in living-related LT or when small-for-size complication is anticipated.

Thrombocytopenia will be aggravated during the surgical procedure due to bleeding and entrapment in the graft secondary to reperfusion. The decrease in platelet number will continue in the initial postoperative phase but a spontaneous resolution will take place if no complication.

Administration of platelets is not indicated if there is no bleeding or immediate bleeding risk. New emerging therapies like thrombopoietin-receptor agonist will furthermore limit the administration of blood products.

Conflict of interest

No potential conflict of interest.

Author details

Gabriela Droc[1,2]*

*Address all correspondence to: gabidroc@gmail.com

1 University of Medicine and Pharmacy "Carol Davila", Bucharest, Romania

2 Fundeni Clinical Institute, Bucharest, Romania

References

[1] Laffi G, Tarquini R, Marra F. Thrombocytopenia in chronic liver disease: Lessons from transplanted patients. Journal of Hepatology. 2007;**47**:625-629

[2] Mitchell O, Feldman DM, Diakow M, Sigal SH. The pathophysiology of thrombocytopenia in chronic liver disease. Hepatic Medicine: Evidence and Research. 2016;**8**:39-50

[3] Pereboom ITA, Lisman T, Porte RJ. Platelets in liver transplantation: Friend or foe? Liver Transplantation. 2008;**14**:923-931. DOI: 10.1002/lt.21510

[4] Peck-Radosavljevic M. Thrombocytopenia in chronic liver disease. Liver International. 2017;**37**:778-793

[5] Afdhal N, McHutchinson J, Brown R, Jacobson I, Manns M, Poordad F, Weksler B, Esteban R. Thrombocytopenia associated with chronic liver disease. Journal of Hepatology. 2008;**48**: 1000-1007

[6] Pamecha V, Mahansaria SS, Kumar S, Bharathy KGS, Sasturkar SV, Sinha PK, Kumar N, Kumar V. Association of thrombocytopenia with outcome following adult living donor. Liver Transplantation. 2016;**29**:1126-1113

[7] Massoud OI, Zein NN. The effect of Transjugular intrahepatic Portosystemic shunt on platelet counts in patients with liver cirrhosis. Gastroenterology & Hepatology. 2017;**13**: 286-291

[8] Gangireddy V, Kanneganti P, Sridhar S, Talla S, Coleman T. Management of thrombocytopenia in advanced liver disease. Canadian Journal of Gastroenterology & Hepatology. 2014;**28**:558-564

[9] Tripodi A, Primignani M, Chantarangkul V, Clerici M, Dell'Era A, Fabris F, et al. Thrombin generation in patients with cirrhosis: The role of platelets. Hepatology. 2006;**44**: 440-445

[10] Saner FH, Gieseler RK, Akiz H, Canbay A, Gorlinger K. Delicate balance of bleeding and thrombosis in end-stage liver disease and liver transplantation. Digestion. 2013;**88**: 135-144

[11] Ohira M, Ishifuro M, Ide K, Irei T, Tashiro H, Itamoto T, Ito K, Chayama K, Asahara T, Ohdan H. Significant correlation between spleen volume and thrombocytopenia in liver transplant patients: A concept for predicting persistent thrombocytopenia. Liver Transplantation. 2009;**15**:208-215

[12] Morimoto H, Ishiyama K, Ishifuro M, Ohira M, Ide K, Tanaka Y, Tahara H, Teraoka Y, Yamashita M, Abe T, Hashimoto S, Hirata F, Tanimine N, Saeki Y, Shimizu S, Sakai H, Yano T, Tashiro H, Ohdan H. Clinical efficacy of simultaneous Splenectomy in liver transplant recipients with hepatitis C virus. Transplantation Proceedings. 2014;**46**:770-773

[13] Chu HC, Hsieh CB, Hsu KF, Fan HL, Hsieh T, Chen T. Simultaneous splenectomy during liver transplantation augments antiviral therapy in patients infected with hepatitis C virus. The American Journal of Surgery. 2015;**209**:180-186

[14] Ito K, Akamatsu N, Ichida A, Ito D, Kaneko J, Arita J, Sakamoto Y, Hasegawa K, Kokudo N. Splenectomy is not indicated in living donor liver transplantation. Liver Transplantation. 2016;**22**:1526-1535

[15] Juttner B, Brock J, Weissig A, Becker T, Studzinski A, Asthaus WA, Bornscheuer A, Scheinichen D. Dependence of platelet function on underlying liver disease in orthotopic liver transplantation. Thrombosis Research. 2009;**124**:433-438

[16] Droc G, Popescu M, Filipescu D, Bubenek S, Popescu I. Defining risk factors for post liver transplant thrombocytopenia. Archives of the Balkan Medical Union. 2015;**50**:309-313

[17] Lesurtel M, Raptis DA, Melloul E, Schlegel A, Oberkoffer C, El-Badry AM, Weber A, Mueller N, Dutkowski P, Clavien PA. Low platelet counts after liver transplantation predict early posttransplant survival: The 60-5 criterion. Liver Transplantation. 2014;**20**: 147-155

[18] Bachmann R, Bachmann J, Lange J, Nadalin S, Konigsrainer A, Ladurner R. Incidence of heparin-induced thrombocytopenia type II and postoperative recovery of platelet count in liver graft recipients. Journal of Surgical Research. 2014;**186**:429-435

[19] Chang FY, Singh N, Gayaowski T, Wagener M, Mietzner S, Stout J, Marino I. Thrombocytopenia in liver transplant recipients: Predictors, impact on fungal infections and role of endogenous thrombopoietin. Transplantation. 2000;**69**:70-75

[20] Stanca CM, Fiel MI, Aledort L, Cohen E, del Rio Martin J, Schiano TD, Factors associated with persistent thrombocytopenia after liver transplantation, Transplantation Proceedings. 2010;**42**:1769-1773

[21] Nascimbe A, Iannacone M, Brando B, De Gasperi A, Acute thrombocytopenia after liver transplant: role of platelet activation, thrombopoietin deficiency and response to high dose intravenous IgG treatment, Journal of Hepatology. 2007;**47**:651-657

[22] Lisman T, Porte RJ. Mechanisms of platelet-mediated liver regeneration. Blood. 2016; **128**:625-629

[23] De Boer MT, Christensen MC, Asmussen M, van der Hilst CS, Hendricks HGD, Sloff MJH, Porte LJ. Impact of intraoperative transfusion of platelets and red blood cells on survival after liver transplantation. Anesthesia and Analgesia. 2008;**106**:32-44

[24] Fayed NA, Abdallah AR, Khalil MK, Marwan IK. Therapeutic rather than prophylactic transfusion policy for severe thrombocytopenia during liver transplantation. Platelets. 2014;**25**:576-586

[25] Pereboom ITA, de Boer MT, Haagsma EB, Hendricks HGD, Lisman T, Porte RJ. Platelet transfusion during liver transplantation is associated with increased postoperative mortality due to acute lung injury. Anesthesia and Analgesia. 2009;**108**:1083-1091

[26] Kim J, Yi NJ, Shin WY, Kim T, Lee KU, Suh KS. Platelet transfusion can be related to liver regeneration after living donor liver transplantation. World Journal of Surgery. 2010;**34**:1052-1058

[27] De Pietri L, Ragusa F, Deleuterio A, Begliomini B, Serra V. Reduced transfusion during OLT by POC coagulation management and TEG functional fibrinogen: A retrospective observational study. Transplantation Direct. 2015. DOI: 10.1097/TXD.0000000000000559 eCollection 2016 Jan

[28] Taura P, Martinez-Palli G, Blasi A, Rivas E, Beltran J, Balust J. Intraoperative management of high risk liver transplant recipients: Concerns and challenges. Transplantation Proceedings. 2016;**48**:2491-2494

[29] Afdhal NH, Giannini EG, Tayyab G, Mohsin A, Lee JW, Andriulli A, Jeffers L, McHutchinson J, Chen PJ, Han KH, Campbell F, Hyde D, Brainsky A, Theodore D, for the ELEVATE study Group. Eltrombopag before procedures in patients with cirrhosis and thrombocytopenia. New England Journal of Medicine. 2012;**367**:716-724